Palliative Care Perspectives

Palliative Care Perspectives

JAMES L. HALLENBECK, M.D.

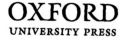

OXFORD
UNIVERSITY PRESS

2003

OXFORD
UNIVERSITY PRESS

Oxford   New York
Auckland   Bangkok   Buenos Aires   Cape Town   Chennai
Dar es Salaam   Delhi   Hong Kong   Istanbul   Karachi   Kolkata
Kuala Lumpur   Madrid   Melbourne   Mexico City   Mumbai
Nairobi   São Paulo   Shanghai   Taipei   Tokyo   Toronto

Copyright © 2003 by Oxford University Press, Inc.

Published by Oxford University Press, Inc.
198 Madison Avenue, New York, New York 10016
http://www.oup-usa.org

Oxford is a registered trademark of Oxford University Press

Library of Congress Cataloging-in-Publication Data

Hallenbeck, James.
Palliative care perspectives / James L. Hallenbeck.
p. ; cm.   Includes bibliographical references and index.
ISBN 978-0-19-516577-7 (cloth); 978-0-19-516578-4 (pbk.)

1. Palliative treatment.   2. Terminal care.   3. Physician and patient.
I. Title.
[DNLM: 1. Palliative Care—methods.
2. Attitude to Death.
3. Pain—therapy.
4. Physician-Patient Relations.
WB 310 H184p 2003]   R726.8 H347 2003   616'.029—dc21   2002042542

Printed in the United States of America
on acid-free paper

For my daughter, Mika

Preface

The purpose of today's training is to defeat yesterday's understanding.

Miyamoto Musashi, Japanese sword master

I never set out to be a palliative care physician. I had tried my hand at being an administrator, but it did not work out. I quit my job coordinating outpatient clinics and began looking for something else to do. As luck would have it, a job just then opened up in a nursing home that had a small inpatient hospice unit. That seemed interesting, I thought, rather dispassionately. I had no idea how radically my life was about to change.

My new job was to begin in January 1994. In December I was scheduled to attend on an academic medical service. I had attended many times before and considered myself an old hand at the job. The work of attending requires a delicate balance. Attending physicians are supposed to know what is going on with the patients on the team and yet leave enough "space" for resident physicians to learn from doing. Done well, attending means providing guidance, wisdom, and humor—setting a tone for the team that is serious without being heavy. Done poorly, it means doing time—a series of canned talks for the team, card-flipping with the residents as to how Mr. or Mrs. Smith is doing, and writing "see and agree" notes that meet the bare minimum requirement for supervision.

As I began my familiar work of attending that month, I was thinking ahead to my future job in hospice. I had been taught virtually nothing about end-of-life care in medical school or residency. Of course, I had cared for my share of dying patients, pronounced a reasonable number of people dead, and treated most common symptoms in some fashion. However, as I faced the prospect of doing hospice, I came to realize how ill-prepared I really was, so I read a little bit during that month. I also tried to see my patients, many of whom happened to be dying, with new "hospice eyes."

I remember one patient in particular. She was a woman with advanced metastatic breast cancer. The resident told me she was in great pain both physically and emotionally. She was on a large dose of morphine, but that did not seem to take care of the problem. She had pneumonia, which was being treated. No one was quite sure what, but there was some issue with her son. We would do what we could. As soon as the antibiotics were finished, she was scheduled to be transferred out—to a nursing home or hospice I cannot remember.

How sad, I thought, as I headed out on my rounds to meet the patients. I imagined the note I would write, "A 74 y.o. woman with metastatic cancer and pneumonia. Patient seen and chart reviewed. Agree with housestaff work-up and plans." I had done it many times before. This time, I paused. This was the kind of patient I would soon be caring for on a regular basis. Perhaps it would be interesting to just sit and talk with her for a while. Perhaps I could learn something about what I was to encounter as a hospice physician.

I approached her, introduced myself, and, with some effort, found a seat. This unusual behavior evoked a scowl from Mrs. B. "What could *you* want," she seemed to ask. To my surprise I thought to myself, "I'm not sure." I was so used to going to the bedside with a clear reason, an agenda, and now I was not sure I had one. It was a scary but rather liberating feeling to approach a patient this way. "I thought we might just talk. I heard from Dr. S. about your situation. It seems like you have been having a hard time." She slowly began to open up. At first she talked about how much her back hurt. Her story then began moving to her relationship with her son. She was very attached to him and worried about how he would manage without her. The depth of her psychic pain seemed to draw in the very light from the room. This was getting heavy and I wanted to back off. Just then, a ray of sunlight came through the window, highlighting a bouquet of flowers on the bed stand behind Mrs. B. Seeing this, I commented on how beautiful they were. Mrs. B choked and said that they were from her son. Then she literally wailed, "If only I could see them." Suddenly, it became clear. Flowers delivered per routine to a hospital patient had been placed, without thinking, in the one place Mrs. B. could never look. Her back pain prevented her from turning toward this precious gift, just as her illness kept her from her son—both out of sight but never out of mind. I rose and moved the flowers to a spot where she could see them. I did not know it at the time, but in retrospect I believe that was the first time I entered the world of hospice.

My memory of the first several months working at my new job in the nursing home is a blur. I had visited a nursing home once or twice before in my life. Overnight I had inherited 75 patients with advanced chronic illness. I was completely unprepared. My friends now tell me they thought I was depressed or, more likely, disgusted by what I saw. I was neither. I was terrified. In arrogance I thought I was a reasonably well-trained internist and that my prior experience would more than suffice. After all, I had been a chief resident at a top flight residency program and had run an intensive care unit, an emergency room, and a general medical clinic. These patients were not even acutely ill, yet I was truly, completely unprepared. Yes, I knew how to prescribe many necessary medicines, but this was such a small part of what these patients needed. Each was struggling in his or her own way with how, simply, to get through the day. Pain, constipation, confusion, diaper rash, immobility, memory loss, depression, and boredom—these and a host of other afflictions beset them. If called upon to kill a wayward pneumococcus with an antibiotic, I was as good as any physician, but in addressing the various miseries associated with chronic illness, I was grossly incompetent.

In the hospital, when I was out of my league it was easy to get a consult. Abnormal antimitochondrial antibody? No problem—a rheumatology consult would explain it all. However, here in the nursing home we were largely on our own. We could send patients to clinic, usually by ambulance, if necessary. An appointment might take weeks or months to get. For the very frail or confused, such adventures were a risky business. Patients could get lost or admitted before you knew it. Very few physicians were willing to make a "house call" to the nursing home. For the most part we, staff and patients, were on our own.

Thinking back, I am extremely grateful to everyone for their patience with me. They say I was often seen walking down the hall hunched over with a frown, only to disappear for long periods into my office. "Depressed? Disgusted? He can't take it. *He* won't last long," they must have thought. In fact, I was reading like crazy in my office. I bought texts on geriatrics and what little was available on hospice and palliative care. Mercifully, not too many months before beginning this work, the *Oxford Textbook of Palliative Medicine* had been published. This book was a godsend for me, orders of magnitude better than anything else available. From this book I got a sense of what was really possible. Fear began to turn to excitement. In fact, there was so much that could be done! As excitement grew, so did anger. Why had I not been exposed to any of this before? I had been trained in some of the best programs in the United States, yet here was a major body of knowledge and skills that was not even on the radar screen of those programs.

I found, after my initial terror, that a whole new world of healing had opened up for me. I was particularly drawn to the then small seven-bed hospice I had inherited that was tucked away in the back corner of the nursing home. Quietly and unassumingly, a dedicated group of individuals had been caring for dying patients for well over 10 years prior to my arrival. If I found excitement (and anger) in my work in the nursing home, in hospice I found my passion. Here, the human condition was boiled down to its essential ingredients. Pain, suffering, love, joy, meaning, and despair all appeared in purified forms, conjured upon before the great mirror of death. The nakedness of these human truths demanded a sincere response. Here was real work to do.

When I attended my first hospice meeting as the hospice physician, the team was tightly gathered around a conference table. I sat outside the circle. The nurses, social workers, volunteers, and others actively discussed each patient. I was not expected to participate. They were not opposed, really, it just had never been done. Having a physician was a legal necessity for signing orders. Little else was expected. The real work (and magic) was to be performed by others. Hospice staff seemed pleasantly surprised when I displayed more than a passing interest in the meeting.

As my passion for hospice and palliative care grew, so did an understanding that I had received a great gift. I had "fallen" willy-nilly into an amazing world where, incredibly, I was free to be a healer. This new work required energy and dedication, yet I found joy in being of some help to others. However much I was able to give, I found I received that much more. Determination grew in me to share this world and what I was learning with others. I suspected I was not the only physician frustrated by modern medicine who wanted to find a different way to help. God knows, there was enough suffering to go around, and so, ill prepared as I was, I began to teach.

First, we established a rotation for geriatric fellows in the nursing home. Incredibly, until then our geriatric fellows spent no time in any nursing homes on the general belief that nursing home patients were beyond hope. Then a clerkship was started for medical students. We explored having interns rotate through the nursing home and hospice. At first, there was a concern on the part of the training program that any such rotation would be very unpopular and "hurt us in the match" (the process by which residency programs choose graduating medical students). We were allowed to start the rotation on a trial basis. It was this comment about such a rotation being a potential detriment to the residency that led me to publish an article in the *Journal of Palliative Medicine* that documented the impact of the rotation, which was extremely popular.[1] Now, years later, our program has expanded to 25 beds and become a separate unit in the main hospital building associated with an active consultation team, clinic, and home care program. We have developed a fellowship program for physicians, nurses, and psychologists. The good news is that physicians and other clinicians *do* want to be of help. Not everybody wants to do advanced training and specialize in palliative care, which is, of course, fine; we need all sorts of healers, and most everybody wants to help. Most trainees are very grateful for the opportunity to increase their skills and, frankly, to compensate for their general lack of training in palliative care elsewhere. Based on this experience, I am encouraged that if we provide the right opportunities, clinicians will want to learn palliative care. To paraphrase the movie *Field of Dreams*, "If we build it, they will come."

About This Book

This book is intended for clinicians relatively new to palliative care who want to learn more about core topics in the field. Practical suggestions for approaching certain care issues are presented. Beyond this, I also hope the text will help readers piece together from overtly disparate topics a more coherent picture of palliative care as it is currently evolving. This book evolved out of talks and presentations given to medical students, residents, and fellows trying to learn palliative care fundamentals with me over the past nine years. As such, the text is probably most appropriate for trainees in similar circumstances. I hope that others, both physicians and nonphysicians, may also find something of use. The text was originally designed to parallel a course given by the Stanford Faculty Development Center in end-of-life care. This course presents seven discrete modules: (1) an overview of death and dying in America, (2) pain management, (3) nonpain symptom management, (4) communication, (5) difficult decisions, (6) psychosocial and spiritual aspects of care, and (7) issues relating to venues of care. The last module also addresses how the clinician can work as an agent of change to improve the quality of palliative care in his or her health care system. Not all topics addressed in the course are covered in this book, and certain topics are covered here that are not covered in the course.

Over the past several years many fine texts and other educational tools have emerged that deal with palliative care. Why another book? Learners have different styles and may be drawn to different formats. Some may do best with classic textbooks. Some may prefer interactive multimedia presentations or problem-based learning. In this book I attempt to be clear but not comprehensive; this is not a textbook, nor is it a simple "how-to" manual. Excellent examples of these types of texts exist, and I do not wish to write another one. I am striving to make some sense of palliative care as I have come to understand it—via *stories*. While I sometimes highlight issues with stories of people, most of these stories attempt to make sense of certain aspects of palliative care. Many stories emerge from core questions about the nature of what we do, such as *why* are we doing such a poor job caring for very sick and dying people and *what* is the relation of hospice to palliative care. While some stories address "big-picture" issues such as these, others are quite practical in their implications. It is often helpful in learning how to treat certain symptoms to make stories about some otherwise complicated pathophysiology and then devise related strategies for treatment. The complex mechanisms of nausea, for example, can best be understood if we first think about *why* we experience nausea and vomiting, which leads to a discussion of the pathophysiology of nausea and finally suggestions for treatment. I combine big-picture issues and nitty-gritty aspects of palliative care in this text because, frankly, both are necessary for good practice. Simple how-to manuals risk reducing the practice of palliative care to recipes, when, in fact, all of us, patients, families, and clinicians, are struggling with big-picture questions when encountering suffering and death. On the other hand, philosophy divorced from practice is a weak brew. Suffering manifests itself concretely in specific pains and agonies that must be addressed in very practical ways. Thus, certain how-to skills will also be discussed within the contexts of particular stories.

Throughout the text I highlight certain points as palliative care notes. Focusing on certain points to the exclusion of others reflects personal biases on my part and even a certain arrogance in directing the reader toward these rules of thumb. For this I ask forgiveness. My hope is that these points will be useful to the reader and serve as guiding principles and, occasionally, as morals to my stories.

We are not so different from our ancestors, who used to sit around campfires telling and hearing stories. People live, learn, and remember through storytelling. The stories presented here reflect my current level of understanding and my efforts to transmit this understanding. While I attempt to provide what evidence I can to support this understanding, for better or worse this text emerges from the thinking and the practice of one palliative care physician. The reader is advised not to accept my writing uncritically. Please do the much needed work for expansion of the evidence base underlying such stories. Test these stories through your practice and your study, and then defeat this level of understanding. In this process I hope you will create new stories to share with others.

Palo Alto, California   J. L. H.

Reference

1. Hallenbeck, J. L. and M. R. Bergen. A medical resident inpatient hospice rotation: Experiences with dying and subsequent changes in attitudes and knowledge. Journal of Palliative Medicine 1999; 2(2): 197–208.

Acknowledgments

I have been very lucky to have found my way to palliative care. As a physician, I feel I have finally found my home in medicine. I am indebted to many individuals who have helped me along the way. To all my teachers, inside and outside of medicine, I offer my gratitude for your patient and kind instruction. To mentors and friends, especially David Weissman, Charles von Gunten, Ira Byock, and Joanne Lynn, and Brad Stuart, thank you for your guidance and role modeling. To the students, residents, and fellows who have crossed my path, it has been a great privilege to work with you. There is no greater joy for a teacher than to see students blossom, becoming teachers in their own right. A special thanks to ex-fellows and good friends Richard Meyers, who helped me in the development of the section on bowel obstruction, and V. J. Periyakoil, who helped in the development of the section on psychosocial issues. To the staff of the Stanford Faculty Development Center, especially Kelley Skeff, Georgette Stratos, Sara Katz, and Jane Mount, thank you for your help in developing our end-of-life care faculty development course. This manual would not otherwise have come into being. I am also indebted to the Robert Wood Johnson Foundation, which in addition to funding the SFDC project, has done so much to further the development of palliative care. Sara Katz, V. J. Periyakoil, Monique Kuo, and Maria Dans are to be thanked for their thoughtful comments and editing of this manuscript. Thank you to Vickii Ellis, Dwight Wilson, and Mark

Graeber for having the foresight to develop the VA Hospice Care Center back in 1979. The hospice you developed is an enduring legacy. I was very fortunate to have been introduced to hospice and palliative care there. My gratitude to the staff and especially the patients and families of the VA Hospice Care Center at the VA Palo Alto Health Care System—on a day-to-day basis you serve as my teachers. Philosophy is grounded in practice, and practice is grounded in community. To have such a wonderful community within which to work is an honor. I am fortunate indeed.

A special thanks to my family, Toriko, Cody, and Mika, for their support. They have had to put up with much over the years. Most especially I must thank my daughter, Mika. She has never said a single word, but she has been my greatest teacher. When I tend to float off in abstract, philosophical fantasies, she brings me down to earth, reminding me that we are all here, together, in the same soup. We are here for each other.

Disclaimer Concerning Medical Information

The information in this book is not medical advice. Health care providers should exercise their own clinical judgment when providing medical care. Some of the information in this manual cites the use of products in dosages for indications in a manner other than that recommended in the product labeling. Accordingly, the official prescribing information should be consulted prior to using any such product. The author is an employee of the Department of Veterans Affairs. This work was written independent of such employment and in no way represents the views or opinions of the Department of Veterans Affairs.

Contents

Palliative Care Perspectives

1

Death and Dying in Modern Times

Young friends regard this solemn Truth, soon you may die like
me in youth: Death is a debt to nature due, which I have paid,
and so must you.

> Tombstone of James Hull Allen, died August 6, 1793,
> age 15 years, 3 months, and 21 days

It's not that I'm afraid to die . . . I just don't want to be there when
it happens.

> Woody Allen, *Without Feathers*

Over the centuries healers have been called upon to palliate, or "make better,"
myriad afflictions. Only in recent times has the notion arisen that our primary
goal is to identify and cure diseases, thereby prolonging life and, presumably,
preventing distressing symptoms and associated suffering. The medical advances
made in recent decades are indeed so astonishing that one could almost forgive
those who would hope that a cure-based medicine might eliminate scourges such
as pain and the debilitations of old age. However, we remain mortal. I recall a
scene from Bernado Bertolucci's film *Little Buddha* in which a child sits with a
wise, old monk looking out over a bustling city in Nepal. "What is impermanence?" asks the child. The monk answers, "See these people. All of us and all
the people alive today. One hundred years from now we'll all be dead. That is

impermanence." Intellectually, I understand the truth of this statement. However, that more than 6 billion people will die in a period of 100 years is beyond my comprehension.

That people die is nothing new. Illness and death have always been part of human experience. Ancient people were plagued by chronic debilitations often associated with parasitic infections.[1] Egyptians in the time of the pharaohs, for example, frequently suffered from schistosomiasis, resulting in chronic pain and weakness. However, how we get sick today and how our society responds to sickness has changed radically. As the nature of illness has changed, so too has dying.[2-5] In 1900 the top five causes of death in the United States were respiratory infections (influenza and pneumonia), tuberculosis, gastroenteritis, heart disease, and stroke, in that order.[6] With the exception of tuberculosis, most other deaths were relatively sudden, occurring over a few days of illness. In 2000 the top five causes of death in the United States were heart disease, cancer, stroke, chronic obstructive pulmonary disease (COPD), and accidents.[7] With the exception of sudden heart attacks and accidental deaths, most of these deaths were due to prolonged, chronic illnesses. While significant differences remain between developed and developing countries in terms of causes of death, the trend seems irreversible: illnesses and deaths associated with infectious and parasitic causes are on the wane, and chronic, degenerative illnesses such as cancer and dementia are increasing.* In 1990 it was estimated that for every death due to cancer worldwide, two deaths occurred due to infectious and parasitic causes. By 2015 this ratio will be one-to-one.[8]

Dying of cholera or some other horrible gastrointestinal scourge seems a very unpleasant way to go. However, because we remain mortal, to prevent one way of dying is, in effect, to "create" another. Even very good things like seatbelts are "carcinogenic" in that by decreasing the chance of dying in car accidents, seatbelts proportionately increase the probability of growing older and dying from other diseases such as cancer. That we are more likely to die of chronic illness at an advanced age is not such a terrible thing, considering the alternatives. However, we must take responsibility for these new forms of illness and associated dying.

This book has an unavoidable bias based on my experience practicing palliative care in the United States. I hope this perspective is not entirely irrelevant to people in other parts of the world who are struggling with illness, death, and suffering. Each society and culture will have its particular issues and challenges. For developing, often impoverished, countries, simply increasing the availability of oral morphine for patients dying of cancer or AIDS may be an overwhelming challenge. Developed countries may be struggling with complex social forces that result in the warehousing of their sickest and dying members in dehuman-

---

*HIV disease is a sad exception.

izing institutions far from family and friends. Despite the great social, cultural, and political differences that divide the globe, I would argue that we have more in common than not. These dramatic changes in how we experience illness and death affect virtually all of us. While we may find guidance and strength in our cultural traditions, I think none of us can rely on old ways of "doing" illness and dying. Cultural traditions related to illness and healing evolved slowly over millennia and are resistant to change. Civilizations developed elaborate ways for dealing with illness. However, as recently as 50 years ago, few people lived to an advanced age. Virtually nobody experienced prolonged states of severe incapacitation and dependence. For most, dying was a brief affair, usually lasting a few days and requiring simple acts of kindness from family and friends.

It is safe to say that our new ways of becoming ill and dying have swamped our cultural coping mechanisms. We are simply unprepared for the vast numbers of people in both developed and developing countries who will succumb to diseases such as cancer, AIDS, and dementia. We must create new ways of responding to modern forms of illness and dying if we are to maintain any hope of living and dying well.

Palliative care, as an international movement, is trying to respond to these changes. Palliative care seeks to use the powerful tools developed by modern medicine to address the needs of the sick in terms of relieving suffering and enhancing quality of life. We must also be mindful that the very same medical system that creates these tools too often creates new forms of suffering that must be addressed. Thus, palliative care must walk a tight-rope—we try to use a system of medicine for the good of patients and families without being overrun and dominated by that system. Only time will tell if we will succeed. The origins of the palliative care movement are to be found in the hospice movement, an alternative approach to dealing with terminal illness.

Hospice Care—Early History

Traditions of kindness for sick and dying patients are to be found in all societies from antiquity. The beginning of the modern hospice movement is usually attributed to Dame Cicely Saunders, who founded St. Christopher's Hospice in London in 1967.[9] Two years later Elizabeth Kübler-Ross published her landmark book, *On Death and Dying*, based on her experiences talking with dying patients in a Chicago hospital.[10] Was it a coincidence that these two landmark events occurred in such close temporal proximity? I do not think so.

In 1953 the first advanced mammal, a dog named Knowsy (because he knew what was on the "other side") was successfully resuscitated.[11] Further advances in resuscitation and advanced life-support led to the propagation of cardiopulmonary resuscitation (CPR) and intensive care units during the early 1960s. Early articles on CPR reflected a naïve optimism and lack of concern for the possible consequences of resuscitation. The development of CPR and advanced life-support was symbolic of much broader changes in how we understand illness and the role of medicine. The goal of medicine shifted from *healing* to *cure*, or the elimination of disease. Given early successes in curing such diseases as pneumococcal pneumonia with penicillin, people began to believe that *everything* could be cured—a "cult of cure" of sorts.[12] The trick seemed to be to break down the human body as a machine into its constituent parts and then figure out how to keep all the parts working or, when irrevocably damaged, how to replace the broken parts. Then, if we knew and could fix all the parts in theory, our body-machines could live on forever. Great idea. Unfortunately, things did not quite work out that way. People grew old, developing aches, pains, and debilitations that the new system of medicine seemed incapable of addressing. Clinicians also become frustrated. Patients, once "fixed," did not stay fixed—they kept bouncing back to the hospital. Somewhere, there was a big mistake.

In retrospect, it seems inevitable that a backlash to such blind optimism would arise. Cicely Saunders and Kübler-Ross, as pioneers, were remarkable in having recognized the mistake far before the rest of us did. It was easiest to recognize the mistake in considering those patients who were overtly dying, yet the power of belief in the cult of cure was (and still too often is) so strong that it denied the very existence of dying patients as a class of people. Deaths, if they occurred, were aberrations; in the cult of cure people did not die, they coded. Kübler-Ross wrote that the greatest barrier to her initial request to speak with dying patients in the hospital was a broad denial that such patients even existed.[10] Cicely Saunders's experiences as a nurse, social worker, and physician convinced her that dying patients were often neglected and ignored, suffering unnecessarily for want of both basic symptom management and attention. A new social institution was needed. This institution became known as hospice.

Early hospices arose as sanctuaries from traditional hospitals.[4,13] The first hospices in North America were founded in 1975 in Connecticut, New York, and Montreal.[14] They were all inpatient units, operating on grants and contributions. In 1979 a hospice was started in Marin, California. That same year the VA Palo Alto Health Care System started a small three-bed inpatient hospice within its newly built nursing home in Menlo Park, California, making it one of the first publicly funded hospices in the country. That hospice evolved into the VA Hospice Care Center, where I currently work. All such early hospices were inpatient facilities. Home hospice, which for many Americans has become synonymous with hospice, was a later development, spurred on in the United States by the creation of the Medicare Hospice Benefit in 1983. This benefit overtly emphasized the provision of hospice at home and more subtly discouraged the creation of dedicated inpatient hospice facilities. The net result in the United States is over 3000 hospice agencies, which provide the vast majority of their care in the home. Few dedicated inpatient hospice units currently exist in the United States. Inpatient hospices like the VA Hospice Care Center have continued within the Department of Veterans Affairs. Hospice care within the Department of Veterans Affairs has evolved independent of Medicare rules.

The Medicare Hospice Benefit did many wonderful things for dying patients. Most obviously, it provided the first funding mechanism dedicated to end-of-life care. The benefit also pushed clinicians to consider healing beyond the narrow medical paradigm. Support for family as "the unit of care" was emphasized. Bereavement follow-up was mandated as a part of the benefit package. However, the package also contained major flaws. In emphasizing care at home, the benefit seemed to ignore the obvious: the majority Americans die in institutions in either acute care or nursing homes. Paraphrasing the words of bank robber Willy Sutton, hospice did not "go where the money is," where most Americans were dying—acute care hospitals. Hospice care was also narrowly defined as applicable only to dying patients. Begging the obvious, it is not only the imminently dying who wish not to suffer during episodes of illness. A broader concept was needed that could build on the strong base established by the hospice movement to address the needs of the dying and nondying beyond home hospice, a concept that has come to be known as palliative care.

Palliative Care and Palliative Medicine

The root word for palliation in Latin, *palliare*, means to cloak or shield. At a simple level we can imagine that palliation protects people from the ravages of illness. *Palliative care* means different things to different people, and modern definitions are rapidly evolving.* (The World Health Organization (WHO) has defined palliative care as care that "affirms life and regards dying as a normal process, . . . neither hastens nor postpones death, . . . [and] provides relief from pain and other distressing symptoms."[15] The emphasis is on symptom management in the dying, with no effort to prolong or hasten death. This definition appears to be synonymous with a reasonable definition of hospice care, but others may define it differently. Much "palliative" chemotherapy, for example, seems to have as a goal of care tumor response or improved survival, not symptom management. A few years ago I did a Medline search for articles with keywords referring to palliation and non–small cell lung cancer. What were the outcome measures examined in these studies? Without exception, all looked at survival rates and tumor

---

*The modern use of the term *palliative care* is usually attributed to Dr. Balfour Mount, one of the founders of the North American hospice/palliative care movement. Working in French-speaking Montreal, Mount felt the need to coin a new term for hospice, as the French equivalent meant almshouse for the poor and elderly. Cicely Saunders reports that he borrowed the term from palliative radiation therapy.

response rates. None examined symptomatic relief.* (The oncologic meaning of palliative care appears to mean simply noncurative, life-prolonging care. While no one has a patent on this word, the WHO and the oncologic meanings are antithetical in nature; one deals with quality and the other with quantity of life.

A third meaning appears to be evolving. Palliative care attempts to alleviate the misery associated with illness, and not exclusively terminal illness. The emphasis remains on patients with serious, life-limiting, usually chronic illnesses. The American Academy of Hospice and Palliative Medicine provides this definition: "The term *palliative care* originally referred to the care of patients with terminal illnesses, but now refers to the care of patients with life-limiting illnesses, whether or not they are imminently dying."[16] Palliative *medicine* has a somewhat more formal ring to it and is very similar in meaning. It suggests that aspect that is the domain of physicians or the more "medical" aspects of palliative care.[17] In its core curriculum the American Academy of Hospice and Palliative Medicine defines palliative medicine as "the study and management of patients with active, progressive, far advanced disease for whom the prognosis is limited and the focus of care is quality of life.[16] The main palliative care group for physicians in the United States is the American Academy of Hospice and Palliative Medicine. The broader National Hospice Organization (NHO) recently changed its name to the National Hospice and Palliative Care Organization. Many have described modern hospice care as being a subset of palliative care, even though hospice as a social institution predated palliative care.[18]

The Relationship Between Hospice and Palliative Care

Historically, some tension has existed between those working in hospice and those involved in palliative care outside formal hospices.[18] While both groups are trying to improve care for suffering patients and their families, the fears and concerns of the two camps are instructive.

At the risk of oversimplification, some working in hospice have been concerned that palliative care may represent a return to a mechanistic form of medicine. Pain, for example, might become its own *disease* to be cured like any other.[19,20] There is concern that physicians may try to dominate care again, as too often happens in traditional medicine, thereby negating the progress that has been made by clinicians in other disciplines who work in an interdisciplinary fashion.

The counterargument by some in the palliative care movement is that hospice, while wonderful in many regards, has been too narrow in focus, serving

---

*Oncologists are beginning to push at least for inclusion of subjective patient responses, positive and negative, as legitimate outcome measures to be reported in clinical trials.

too few suffering and dying patients. Hospice has become less a philosophy of care and more a social organization of home care. Hospices have been reluctant to address flaws in the Medicare Hospice Benefit in part because home hospices are dependent upon the benefit for their very existence. Historically, hospices in the United States have done a poor job of advocating for physician education and wider availability of good end-of-life care for those unable to die at home.

I believe there is some truth to both sides of the argument. It would be terrible if palliative care became mechanical symptom management—if *suffering* became a *disease*. Those involved in palliative care must keep close to heart the lessons and wisdom that have evolved in the hospice movement lest we succumb to such a fate. There is also truth in the fact that hospice, at least in the United States, has become bureaucratically encrusted and is due for reform.

The tension between hospice and palliative care has been largely productive. Hospices are providing a moral conscience necessary for the modern palliative care movement. In turn, palliative care is invigorating the hospice movement. In the end, I believe both hospices and those involved in palliative care will be stronger and better for this tension and the ensuing debate.

Recent History

The 1990s witnessed remarkable changes in the palliative care/hospice movement. The first major textbook in the field, *The Oxford Textbook of Palliative Medicine*, was published in 1993. This text was a quantum leap beyond earlier handbooks in the field. While initially hospice was made available primarily to cancer patients, patients with other diseases have begun requesting such care. Pressure is growing to build upon what has been learned in hospices and apply this knowledge to the care of other patients and in other venues. Clinicians are finally beginning to realize that their training has been grossly deficient in the skills and the art of palliative care. Perhaps most important, a significant portion of the public has been exposed to hospice. Consumers are demanding better symptom management and better care—whether they are dying or not—in all venues of care. The public is debating the ethics of assisted suicide and pain management. The tide is beginning to turn.

For the physician-in-training the changes are just beginning. Until recently most medical schools and residency programs in the United States offered limited training in palliative care.[21-24] Most medical schools offer some brief exposure to medical ethics, but rarely symptom management. Residents have been expected to learn skills (such as pain management, sharing bad news, and how to pronounce patients) on the job, usually from residents a year or so senior with similarly poor preparation. This is changing. Many accrediting bodies, from the

American Academy of Medical Colleges to the American Board of Internal Medicine, now require some training in palliative care.[25,26] In January 2000 the Joint Commission on Accreditation of Healthcare Organizations (JCAHO), which accredits hospitals in the United States, issued stringent new requirements for symptom management in hospitals, nursing homes, and clinics.[27] California has passed a law requiring all physicians to receive 12 hours of continuing education credit in pain and end-of-life care between 2002 and 2006 in order to be relicensed. While the quantity and quality of such training is still highly variable, the trend seems irreversible. Palliative care is finally on the radar screen.

The Future

Prophecy is a dangerous but necessary business in medicine. What is the prognosis for palliative care over the next several decades? The only thing I can predict with certainty is that we will be surprised. The rapid evolution of palliative care in the past few years is a hopeful sign that we may be able to adapt to the broader societal changes underway in how we age, experience illness, and die. Here, I will tease out of an uncertain future one facet that I believe is relatively clear barring even more radical and unforeseen developments—a significant increase in the numbers of elderly and chronically ill individuals.

Baby boomers are getting old. The year 2010 will see the beginning of a rapid increase in the number of Americans over age 65. In the span of a mere 30 years, by 2030, the number of Americans over age 65 will double from approximately 35 to 70 million.[28] Boomers tended to have fewer children than did their parents. Thus, we can safely predict that not only will there be more elderly people, there will be proportionately fewer younger workers and caregivers to support them. In 1940, when Social Security was first formed in the United States, 41 workers supported one benefit recipient. In 1998 the ratio was 3.4:1, and in 2030 the ratio will be 2.1:1.[29]* (This phenomenon is not isolated to the United States. A recent UN conference estimated that the number of people over age 60 will triple in the coming 50 years to 2 billion, approximately one-third of the world population. As birth rates fall, the numbers of younger people available to work and care for these elders will decrease. Currently, worldwide the proportion of working-age people to retirees is estimated to be 9:1. In 50 years it will be 4:1. In areas strongly affected by the AIDS epidemic such as Africa and Southeast Asia, it is the working-age adults and their children who are being stricken. They are often cared for by working grandparents.[30] When these grandparents become too frail to work, who will care for them? The smaller pool of young and healthy workers will have to dedicate a greater percentage of their labor to the

---

*I am indebted to Ira Byock, who kindly shared these references with me.

care of the older generation. To the children of my generation I can only say, "Work hard; we are going to need all the help we can get."

We can also reasonably predict that for those chronically ill elders in need of significant personal care, there will be fewer family members available to provide it. In part this will result from boomers having fewer children. Our children are more likely to live at a distance than was so in past generations. In most countries women, who historically have disproportionately provided such care, are more likely to be employed and less likely to be willing or able to quit their jobs to care for a sick parent, parent-in-law, or spouse.[31,32]

For the chronically ill who wish to live and die at home, when family members are unavailable to provide such care, the prospect of being able to hire professional aides also appears grim. Already, well before the boomer glut of the aging, there is a shortage of home health workers in America. This work ranks low on the social ladder, with wages just barely above minimum wage, and attracts the disadvantaged—often poorly educated, immigrant, and minority workers. Barring some dramatic change in how this work is publicly reimbursed, which seems unlikely in the short run, severe shortages of home health workers appear inevitable. The provision of care for chronically ill persons will increasingly be a privilege of the rich, who will have to pay large out-of-pocket sums to attract a small pool of workers.

If this prediction is correct, then, contrary to the hopes of many, fewer chronically ill people will be able to receive the care necessary for living at home. Inevitably, this will shift more people into institutional settings. It has been estimated that the number of Americans living in nursing homes will climb from 1.3 million currently to 5.3 million by 2030.[7] If this occurs, a great challenge will be to reform existing institutions such as nursing homes and to create new institutions wherein we can deliver and receive humane care, including good palliative care.

While the above prediction (sadly) seems relatively safe to me, fundamental changes in how we age and become ill could change this situation. Although immortality is unlikely, at least in my lifetime, it does seem possible that recent medical developments may significantly affect the common courses of illnesses. Cancers might be cured. Alzheimer's disease might become preventable and treatable. It even seems possible that we will be able to slow the aging process in fundamental ways. If such changes come to pass, it is possible that fewer elders will need financial or personal support for long periods during old age. We can imagine that elders might remain very healthy into advanced old age until they undergo a rapid deterioration in health (a compression of morbidity into a shorter time span) or they choose to die[33,34] (see Fig. 1.1).

While this seems theoretically possible, history would argue against this scenario; fixing one problem tends to create others. Thus, it would seem dangerously naïve to believe that medical advances over the next 20 to 30 years will

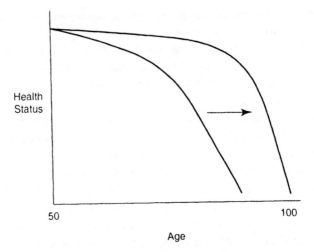

Figure 1.1. Compression of morbidity. The hope expressed in this theory is that various interventions such as healthier lifestyles, preventive medicine, and other medical interventions will shift the curve of decline in health status to the right.

somehow save us from the demographic challenges we face. Assuming we will not be "saved" by a new biomedical revolution, if we do not at least make significant improvements in our health care system to accommodate the growing number of chronically ill, elderly, and dying people, we face disaster. There simply will not be enough nursing home beds, enough workers, or enough money to provide even the most basic care for those who will need it.

References

1. Fabrega, H. *Evolution of Sickness and Healing.* 1997, University of California Press: Berkeley.
2. Cassel, C., ed. *Approaching Death—Improving care at the end of life.* 1997, Institute of Medicine, National Academy Press: Washington, D.C., pp. 33–49.
3. Brock, D. B. and D. J. Foley. Demography and epidemiology of dying in the U.S. with emphasis on deaths of older persons. Hosp J 1998; 13(1–2): 49–60.
4. Kearl, M. *Endings—A Sociology of Death and Dying.* 1989, Oxford University Press: New York, pp. 437–43.
5. Aries, P. *The Hour of Our Death.* 1981, Knopf: New York.
6. Lerner, M. When, why and where people die. In: E. Sneiderman, ed. *Death, Current Perspectives.* 1976, Mayfield: Palo Alto.
7. *Deaths: Preliminary Data for 2000,* vol. 49. 2001, National Center for Health Statistics.
8. Stjernward, J. and S. Pampallona. Palliative medicine—A global perspective. In: D. Doyle, G. Hanks, et al., eds. *Oxford Textbook of Palliative Medicine.* 1998, Oxford University Press: New York, pp. 1227–45.

9. Du Boulay, S. *Cicely Saunders*, 2nd ed. 1994, Hodder & Stoughton: London.
10. Kübler-Ross, E. *On Death and Dying*. 1969, Macmillan: New York.
11. Kouwenhoven, W. The development of the defibrillator. Ann Intern Med 1969; 71: 449–58.
12. Golub, E. *The Limits of Medicine—How Science Shapes Our Hope for the Cure*. 1994, Times Books: New York.
13. Abel, E. K. The hospice movement: Institutionalizing innovation. Int J Health Serv 1986; 16(1): 71–85.
14. Stoddard, S. *The Hospice Movement*. 1992, Vintage: New York.
15. Doyle, D., G. W. C. Hanks, et al. *Oxford Textbook of Palliative Medicine*, 2nd ed. 1998, New York: Oxford University Press, p. 3.
16. Schonwetter, R., ed. *Hospice and Palliative Medicine—Core Curriculum and Review Syllabus*. 1999, Kendall/Hunt: Dubuque, p. 1.
17. Storey, P. and C. F. Knight. *UNIPAC One: The Hospice/Palliative Medicine Approach to End-of-Life Care*. 1998, Kendall/Hunt: Dubuque, p. 11.
18. Byock, I. R. Hospice and palliative care: A parting of ways or a path to the future. Journal of Palliative Medicine 1998; 1(2): 165–75.
19. Kearney, M. Palliative Medicine—Just another specialty? Palliat Med 1992: 6: 39–46.
20. Mann, S. and T. Welk. Hospice and/or palliative care. American Journal of Hospice and Palliative Medicine 1997; 14: 314–5.
21. Dickinson, G. E. Death education in U.S. medical schools: 1975–1980. Journal of Medical Education 1981; 56(2): 111–4.
22. Billings, J. Medical education for hospice care: A selected bibliography with brief annotations. Hospice Journal 1993; 9(1): 69–78.
23. Billings, J. A. and S. Block. Palliative care in undergraduate medical education. Status report and future directions. JAMA 1997; 278(9): 733–8.
24. Hallenbeck, J. L. and M. R. Bergen. A medical resident inpatient hospice rotation: Experiences with dying and subsequent changes in attitudes and knowledge. Journal of Palliative Medicine 1999; 2(2): 197–208.
25. Learning objectives for medical student education—Guidelines for medical schools: Report I of the Medical School Objectives Project. Acad Med 1999; 74(1): 13–8.
26. American Academy of Medical Colleges. *The Increasing Need for End of Life and Palliative Care Education*. Contemporary Issues in Medical Education. 1999, American Academy of Medical Colleges.
27. Joint Commission on Accreditation of Healthcare Organizations. *Pain Standards*. http://www.jcaho.org/standard/stds2001_mpfrm.html, 2001.
28. Fowles, D., A. Duncker, et al. *Profile of Older Americans*. www.aga.gov/aga/stats/profile, 2001.
29. The ghost of Social Security. Editorial *Wall Street Journal* 2000, July 12; A26.
30. Socolovsky, J. Population time bomb: The elderly. *San Francisco Chronicle* 2002; 17.
31. Cline, S. *Lifting the Taboo—Women, Death and Dying*. 1995, New York University Press: New York.
32. Field, D., J. Hockey, et al., eds. *Death, Gender and Ethnicity*. 1997, Routledge: New York.
33. Fries, J. F. Aging, natural death, and the compression of morbidity. N Engl J Med 1980; 303(3): 130–5.
34. Fries, J. F. The compression of morbidity: Near or far? Milbank Q 1989; 67(2): 208–32.

2

Dying Trajectories and Prognostication

"Doc, how much time do I have?" Patient
"Dying? No, I would not say she is dying." Doctor
"Prognosis grim." Note in chart
"Would you be surprised if the patient died in the next two years?"
Dr. Marilyn Patterson
"The operation was successful, but the patient died." Old medical saying/joke

Prognostication, as an art, refers to prediction and communication about future health. Prognostication relates not only to predicting death, but other outcome states such as what percentage of patients with a cancer of a certain stage on initial presentation will eventually develop metastatic disease. As Nicholas Christakis points out, of three traditional domains of medicine (diagnosis, therapy, and prognosis), prognosis has received relatively little attention in modern medical training and research.[1] It is easier to predict when death will occur for patients with some illnesses than for others. Proper prognosis at the end of life enables better decision making about care options and planning for patients and families. The definitive text on prognosis as it relates to palliative care is *Death Foretold: Prophecy and Prognosis in Medical Care* by Christakis.[1]

Predicting Death: The Search for the Holy Grail of Prognosis

We all desire and fear certainty. A desire for certainty arises, I think, in response to apparent chaos in the world.[2,3] However, fear arises because not all that is certain is good. Certainty also negates ambiguity and possibility, wherein people find hope that they can alter a problematic future. Therefore, an intense desire arises for some magic formula that will erase such uncertainty. While people may lament their lack of control over 'bad' outcomes such as death, the ability to predict and know the future represents a form of control if the future unfolds as predicted. Many studies have been devoted to a search for certainty in predicting death, often with little to show for it. It is very disturbing to many that dying is a process largely beyond mortal control.

Prediction of death is *not* linear. That is, we are not necessarily better at predicting death in an ultrashort time frame (seconds to hours) than we are in a long time frame (months to years). Rather, it is like predicting the weather. In California we are good at long-range predictions for a dry summer and wet winter. We are good at predicting that rain will fall on a certain day two to five days beforehand but cannot make such a prediction a month beforehand. In the ultrashort range it defies our abilities to predict *exactly* when the next raindrop will hit a finger. Similarly, we are fairly good at predicting that a patient is at a high risk of dying over a matter of several months. For certain diseases, especially cancer, we are reasonably good at predicting death over a matter of weeks. It is usually impossible to predict the exact moment of death.

Most "holy grail" approaches to predicting death use a grouping of diagnostic criteria and apply them at a certain point in time to establish a probability of dying at some time in the future.[4] The major problem with these approaches is that they are usually discrete, one-time predictions. Real clinical prognostication is more iterative, a form of "fuzzy logic."[5] That is, the most valuable prognostic tool is to note the magnitude of change observed since the last prediction and incorporate this change into a new prediction. For most serious and chronic disease processes the earlier trend of an illness is the best predictor of the future trend. Patients whose clinical decline is rapidly accelerating will likely die sooner than those with otherwise identical clinical parameters but who decline more slowly.

Palliative Care Note

Our most valuable prognostic tool is to note the change observed since our last prediction and incorporate this into our new prediction.

Recent studies have pointed out physician deficits in terms of the ability to predict time of death.[6-8] The general bias in physicians is to be overly optimistic about prognosis by a factor of twofold to fivefold, although errors at the other extreme have also been observed. Christakis and Lamont, in a study of 343 physicians, studied their ability to predict time of death for 468 patients referred to hospice. They found that only 20% of predictions were accurate (within 33% of actual survival), with 63% of predictions overly optimistic and 17% overly pessimistic. Accuracy was calculated by dividing predicted by observed life expectancy. Values falling between .67 and 1.33 were considered accurate. Median life expectancy was 24 days from referral to hospice. On average physicians overestimated life expectancy by a factor of 5. It is interesting to note that 67% of the patients had cancer, usually considered to have a relatively predictable dying trajectory. In this study cancer patients were the most likely to have overly optimistic predictions.[7]

There are many theoretical reasons why physicians are as inaccurate as they appear to be. For a more detailed discussion of these issues the reader is referred to Christakis's book on prognosis. I highlight here only a few key points:

1. Poor predictions may reflect educational deficiencies in clinicians. Because prognosis as a medical art, especially as it relates to dying, has been devalued, better training about what is predictive would likely improve things.
2. Optimistic predictions may reflect a socially sanctioned selection bias for physicians. After all, who wants a pessimist for a doctor? We may select and reward those clinicians who have a rosy view of things.
3. What teaching does exist about prognosis is often gleaned from controlled trials, which tend to carefully select "ideal" patients with isolated diseases, otherwise good health statuses, and thus better prognoses than in patients usually encountered in practice. In cases in which patients have multiple diseases (comorbidities) clinicians may prognosisticate based on each individual disease as a discrete entity, rather than consider how diseases interact in the person to create a particular illness with a poorer prognosis in sum than is implied by consideration of isolated diseases.

Prognosis as a Process of Communication

A very different way to look at prognosis is as a process in communication, central to relationships among clinicians, families, and patients.[9] Families and patients can be greatly helped by an accurate prognosis, but this is not the only relevant issue. Prognostication can be a test of the physician's power; the more accurate the prognosis, the more powerful the "wizard–physician." While patients and families want a powerful physician, they are often conflicted because usually part of them wants the physician to be wrong when it comes to predicting bad things like death. Perhaps if we are wrong as to *when* a patient will die, we might be wrong as to whether the patient really *is* dying. A desire for hope often conflicts with the desire for certainty in prognosis. The physician, as (perceived) keeper of prognostic wisdom, is often a target for the conflicting emotions that arise between the desire for hope and the quest for certainty. Skill is required for safe passage between these extremes.

It is easier to comment on what *not* to say about prognosis at the end of life than on what to say. An almost certain mistake is to tell someone that they will die in X (days, months, years). The odds that the person will actually expire on the appointed day are slim. If death comes earlier, perhaps it may be due to some mistake or oversight on the physician's part. If death comes later, then clearly the physician did not know what he or she was talking about. Either way, the relationship with the physician will be threatened by such inept communication. Equally poor are throw-away line such as "Only God knows." While perhaps true in a literal sense because the *exact* moment of death is unknowable, this is a cop-out with religious trimming.

The trick seems to be to communicate what is and is not known about a patient's prognosis in a manner that strengthens the relationship between physician and patient/family while meeting informational needs. Usually, it is best to give ranges of time for prognoses—hours to days, days to weeks, weeks to months, or months to years. You may need to explain that you are not trying to be vague, but that our ability to predict death is imperfect at best. Rather than set yourself up for a fall with a prediction that may go wrong, your relationship may actually be strengthened by empathizing with the desire for greater certainty. In revealing your humanity and imperfection, you will have found common ground with the patient and family in the face of the mystery of death.* You may need to educate them on exactly *how* you go about telling when someone is about to die by saying, for example, "It helps to know how similar patients with similar illnesses have done, and my prior experience is useful. But most important now, more important than any blood test, is following the trend for your loved one. How he/she progresses over time will help us the most in getting a better reading on when death will come. We'll keep in touch with you as we see how things are changing." Such a statement reflects the iterative process of prognosis and invites ongoing discussion, strengthening the relationship.

Palliative Care Note

Give time estimates for life expectancy in ranges—months to years, weeks to months, days to weeks.

---

*Christakis acknowledges the potential for finding common ground in this manner but concludes that such a use of uncertainty is rare. "Indeed this aspect of prognosis is very unusual in medical practice. This is one area where physicians' revealing their ignorance, uncertainty, fallibility, and vulnerability to patients may have positive effects, helping to build relationships with patients and to humanize physicians in their eyes." (Christakis 1999, p. 60)

Requests for prognosis may relate to very practical needs, such as whether to reschedule a meeting or a trip or a common desire by a loved one to be at the bedside when the person dies. It may be very helpful to inquire *why* someone is asking just then about prognosis rather than assuming you know the answer. This helps frame your response. What they may want, in fact, is a concrete recommendation as to whether the family should be called or a change in plans made. You might want to give more concrete advice on this while admitting uncertainty about the timing of death.

One of the best ways to deal with conflicting desires for certainty and hope in prognosis is to bring the inquirer into the discussion; do not just answer the question. You might ask how much time he or she feels the patient has. An empathetic inquiry can go a long way in dealing with the stress of uncertainty. For example, "It must be hard sitting by the bedside, day after day. How are you doing—are you taking care of yourself?" I have also found it useful sometimes to ask patients themselves how much time they feel they have when discussing prognosis. Some patients seem to express this communication as a "message" from their body. "My body is telling me that it is dying." Thus, I may ask, "What is your body telling you about how much time you have (or more ambiguously, how you are doing)?" Such a question, while admittedly confusing to some patients, can help get patients out of a more abstract conceptualization as to when they might *like* to die into the experience of dying. The question may also help patients pay attention to messages from their bodies they may be ignoring.

Our prognoses will never be perfect. There will always be mystery regarding exactly when people die (and why). However, we can recognize certain patterns of dying that can help us better prognosticate and communicate about dying.

Dying Trajectories

The concept of a dying trajectory was first suggested by Glaser and Strauss in 1965 and refers to the change in health status over time as a patient approaches death.° [13] It is usually plotted (retrospectively for an individual) with time on the X axis and health status on the Y axis. Sudden death has the simplest graph, a

---

°Glaser and Strauss identified different "patterns" of dying—sudden death, lingering, certain to die on time, and the vacillating pattern. Their focus was on expectations about when a patient would die and communication among hospital staff, patients, and families regarding such expectations. The first to use the term *dying trajectory* may have been Gustafson in an article referring to the "careers" of nursing home patients in terms of such trajectories. [10] Shneidman, in a book published shortly after this, explicitly uses the term *death trajectories* relative to the expected time until death. [11] Formally plotting dying trajectories as health status over a longer period of time and considering systemic implications of different trajectories appears to have been the creation of Joanne Lynn and colleagues relative to the very famous SUPPORT study. [12]

rectangle with a straight line down from a state of being healthy to death. The concept of dying trajectories has been helpful in understanding patterns of advanced illness and dying for different disease processes, which, in turn, have implications for care needs, decision making, and prognostication. Individuals will, of course, vary in their personal dying trajectories; however, it is remarkable how similar dying trajectories can be for patients with similar disease processes. Here I will discuss certain common trajectories and their implications.

Sudden Death

The person found suddenly and unpredictably dead is technically beyond the care of the physician (Fig. 2.1). However, survivors are not. It is often the physician who must notify others and provide initial support. Physicians also must provide healthcare to those who have been so bereaved (see section on bereavement in Chapter 7). People may die suddenly and peacefully but more commonly die from accidents or violence, especially the young. The hallmark of this trajectory is lack of preparation for dying. Usually, those who die, unless already very ill or of advanced age, will not have prepared for their death. Even if details such as wills and funeral plans have been made, they have often not had a chance to settle matters in their minds or say goodbye, nor have their loved ones. In addition to the shock of sudden separation and bereavement, survivors may have regrets or feel guilty that they did something wrong or should have done or said something different. Bereavement needs are intense, especially for those bereaved of the young or through violence. Incredibly, many health care sys-

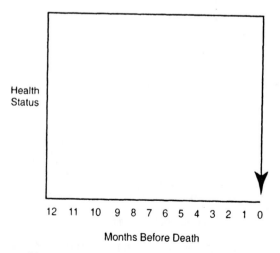

Figure 2.1. Sudden death trajectory.

tems that deal with sudden death have not established even rudimentary support systems for those in need.

Cancer Deaths

Cancers of very different tumor types and locations often follow very similar dying trajectories (Fig. 2.2). In fact, the dying trajectory of cancer is one of the most predictable trajectories. Most patients with metastatic cancer remain quite functional until approximately five to six months before their deaths. Their health statuses then tend to slowly decline until the rate of decline begins to accelerate rapidly two to three months before death.[14] In Teno's study one month prior to death more than 50 percent of the 1655 cancer patients studied had difficulty getting out of a bed or chair. Prior to the period of decline in the last few months of life, cancer patients may have various symptom needs such as pain management but tend to remain at high functional levels. During the rapid decline phase patients start to "take to their beds." A good rule of thumb is that a patient with advanced cancer who has taken to bed *without a correctable cause* will usually die in a matter of weeks to a few months. (*Usually* means *usually*, as I have treated many patients who are exceptions to this rule of thumb.) The caveat about correctable causes is important. Treating certain very responsive cancers with chemotherapy can get people out of bed. Treating complications such as certain infections sometimes makes a difference. This rapid decline in functional status in the last few weeks to months of life correlates highly with admission to and life expectancy in hospice. Christakis in 1996 identified a median survival

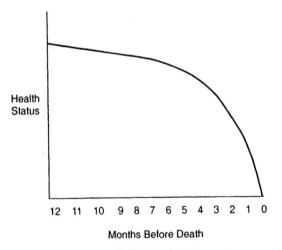

Figure 2.2. Cancer dying trajectory after Teno. In Teno's study health status was measured by age-adjusted activities of daily living (ADL) scores.[15]

of 36 days for 6451 patients followed on the Medicare hospice benefit. Eighty percent of these patients had cancer.[7]

Palliative Care Note

Patients with advanced cancer who have taken to bed *without a correctable cause* will usually die in a matter of weeks to months.

Hospice care, as initially envisioned by Cicely Saunders, was developed primarily with this dying trajectory in mind, and it works rather well for cancer patients, as their deaths are relatively predictable once this decline begins. Prior to the rapid decline phase in the last few weeks to months, it may be very hard to predict when patients with certain cancers will die. Patients with metastatic prostate, breast, and colon cancer, for example, may live for years prior to declining. Many cancer patients do not really *need* home hospice care in the months prior to the accelerated period of rapid decline; their symptoms can be adequately managed on office visits, and psychosocial concerns may be addressed in different ways such as through support groups.

What are the implications of this dying trajectory? When the rapid decline phase begins, prediction of death in a matter of weeks to months is considerably more certain than for most other diseases. With accurate prognostication by the clinician, patients really can know that they will likely die soon. This may come as a surprise, despite having known and even accepted their terminal diagnoses. Patients and families usually have not been taught about this trajectory, and thus, when rapid decline begins, they are often shocked and say, "But he was just fine a couple of weeks ago." Frequently, there is a push to do something to reverse the course of decline. Patients, families, and physicians may be drawn into a frantic dance, which does little but reassure everyone that "everything was tried." This dying trajectory, if recognized, offers the potential for getting one's house in order. Clear prognostication can grant patients and families the time and the permission to take care of unfinished business and to say their goodbyes. For many this is a valuable gift.

Sine-Waving

Congestive heart failure (CHF), chronic obstructive pulmonary disease (COPD), strokes, and many infirmities of advanced age follow a very different pattern (Fig. 2.3).[14] The overall health status of the patient is low 6 to 24 months prior to death. Acute exacerbations of illness (episodes of pulmonary edema, COPD flare-ups, aspiration pneumonias) occur intermittently and tend to increase in frequency until patients often appear to be "sine-waving" (oscillating from chronic ill health to acute crisis).[15] Such patients, if being treated in the hospital, will

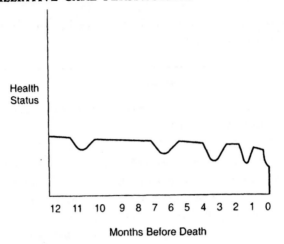

Figure 2.3. Sine-wave dying trajectory.

usually have two to three or more admissions for such exacerbations in the year prior to death. Compared to patients with cancer, it is generally much more difficult to predict death within a matter of weeks to months.[16-18]

Clinicians often will not identify patients with serious, life-limiting illnesses as having terminal illnesses and thus may delay necessary discussions. If asked if such patients are dying, many clinicians will say "no." However, if asked, "Would you be *surprised* if such a patient were to die in the next two years," clinicians will tend to say they would not be surprised.° While such patients may or may not qualify for hospice, they have special care needs, and their dying trajectory has important implications for decision making.

Palliative Care Note

If you would not be surprised if a patient were to die in the next two years, that patient has a *serious, life-limiting illness* and would likely benefit from serious discussion and planning relative to end-of-life care.

This trajectory is extremely common. Patients are at risk of bouncing back and forth from home or nursing home to the hospital, on and off antibiotics, into and out of crisis. House staff in a given hospital often know these patients by name. They are the "frequent fliers." They are particularly troublesome to phy-

---

°This now famous question, "Would you be surprised if the patient died in the next two years," was brought to the attention of the palliative care community by Joanne Lynn in her publications.[19] The first person to use this question as a means of identifying patients with serious, life-threatening illnesses was Dr. Marilyn Patterson, a colleague of Dr. Lynn (personal communication).

sicians and the health care system because they do not behave as they should. Once "fixed," they do not stay fixed. Only with tongue in cheek can the discharge summary conclude, "The patient was stabilized and discharged to home." Patients and families entering this trajectory frequently live miserably on a roller coaster of decline and transient improvement.

This trajectory often can be recognized only after several such episodes of decline. Even so, there is no guarantee that the next dip on the ride will be the last one. Patients, families, and physicians, while despising the seemingly endless cycle of decline and improvement, often act as if they are addicted to it. Even knowing that one more transfusion will not make a difference or that one more round of antibiotics or one more trip to the intensive care unit (ICU) will not help, many have trouble breaking the cycle.

People have trouble accepting the inherent uncertainty in this trajectory. They want to know for sure when death will come—that is, be sure that one more round of therapy will not work. Patients may ask me, "But Doc, the antibiotics got me through the last pneumonia, how do you know they won't work the next time?" We do not, and that is the problem. To deal with this dying trajectory, patients, families, and clinicians must accept prognostic uncertainty and incorporate such uncertainty into their decision making. The question for such patients may be less about how *long* they will live and more about *how* and *where* they wish to live until they do die at some point in an uncertain future.

This trajectory also highlights a problem that can also occur on the cancer trajectory and subsequent trajectory. Will care be defined by what will be done or what will not be done? If clinicians approach patients and families and recommend that no antibiotics be given, blood no longer be transfused, no more admissions to the ICU be authorized, no more IVs or tube feeding be administered, addressing only what will not be done . . . , is it any wonder that they recoil? Here I offer a clinical pearl, nobody is going to love you for what you *do not* do. If only treatment limitation or withdrawal is discussed, patients and families will understandably feel abandoned. Reasonable and caring *alternatives* must be offered. The clinician must be able to say what *will* be done. A weak statement such as "We'll try to keep you comfortable," is not good enough. Unfortunately, many clinicians are ill-prepared to discuss alternatives.

Palliative Care Note

Nobody is going to love you for what you do not do.

Patients on this trajectory face complex choices: where to live (home, assisted living, nursing home, palliative care unit), under what care arrangements (family support, home care, hospice care, etc.), and with what goals of care (comfort only, intermediate life-prolonging efforts, or maximal life-prolonging efforts).

The complexity of such choices makes it tempting for patients, families, and physicians to ignore such choices and to hope that the problem will solve itself. It will eventually, but often at too high a price. One of the most difficult tasks in palliative care, requiring great communication skills in addition to a solid knowledge base about reasonable options, is helping patients and families sort through the complex maze of choices patients encounter on this trajectory.

Deaths Following Aggressive Life-Sustaining Treatment in Acute Care

This dying trajectory is common to many illnesses; patients may have chronic illnesses with sine-waving (see above) or may suffer acute, catastrophic events, such as stroke, overwhelming sepsis, or adverse outcomes of surgery.[20] What characterizes this trajectory is that despite aggressive treatment, the patient does not improve and continues to decline. Many patients will die while such aggressive care continues. The probability of imminent death may not be recognized by patients, families, or health care workers. For others a point comes at which there is recognition that further aggressive, life-sustaining care is very unlikely to be successful, and death can be anticipated in minutes to days.

When impending death has *not* been recognized, the actuality of death often comes as a shock to families and health care workers. These patients do not die, they "code." The emotional impact of such deaths can be great. While families and physicians may experience some satisfaction in that "everything was tried," second thoughts and guilt also commonly arise. "Was there some mistake made?" "What else could have been done?" "Should we have seen this coming?" Patients who die in this way are usually heavily enmeshed in complex, high-tech medicine, and early grief reactions of patients, families, and clinicians may focus on the appropriateness or inappropriateness of specific medical therapies. In bereavement, grief may dwell on missed opportunities, especially if, in retrospect, it should have been clear that the patient was dying.

When death is predicted, a different challenge arises. In most such cases the patient's death will occur in the not-distant future, regardless of specific care decisions. Nevertheless, a myriad of care decisions present themselves to clinicians and families (and occasionally patients), usually relating to treatment withdrawal. Should ICU care, pressors, intubation, antibiotics, dialysis, and so on be withdrawn? Secondarily, parties may discuss where the patient should go following such withdrawal (to the floor, nursing home, home, hospice). In such situations families and clinicians frequently feel an overwhelming sense of responsibility. It is no small thing to discontinue life support and see a patient die soon thereafter. These difficult decisions beset families at a time when they are heavily grieving the impending loss of a loved one. Special communication skills are needed to help families at such times. (See Chapter 8 on Communication) At times families may have trouble experiencing this grief directly, as their energy is consumed with one medical decision after another. Grief becomes walled-off and delayed, risking more intense bereavement later.

Patients on this trajectory often move abruptly from aggressive, life-prolonging efforts to care focused on comfort, a process often called treatment withdrawal. I hate the term. It suggests that care goes from something to nothing. I hate it more when this is, in fact, the case. Statements such as "There is nothing more we can do" reflect such a mindset. I prefer to think of it as a shift or transition in the focus of care. It may be perfectly reasonable to go full-bore trying to save a person's life and equally reasonable to shift that intensity and energy into supporting the patient and the family when it is recognized that dying is happening.[21]

Even when excellent palliative care is available, patients and families on this trajectory often do experience a form of withdrawal. "Detoxification" is required. They have grown accustomed to being cared for through high-tech medicine. Strange as it may seem, having one's blood pressure or O_2 saturation measured may be a way of being nurtured. Suddenly, *not* having tests or vital signs taken can be experienced as abandonment, even when there is no rational reason for continuing such procedures. Thus, careful explanation is needed for why certain things are not being done and why others may be required, even when one might think the reasoning is obvious. New forms of nurturing must be identified.

Finally, a peculiar boomerang effect may be experienced with this trajectory. Having pushed very hard to prolong life and having heard that the patient will soon die, there may arise an expectation or even a desire that death happen very soon after a shift in the focus of care. Some deaths do soon follow, but not always. The reasons for a desire for a quick death are complex. First, having come to recognize dying, there is commonly an understandable desire not to draw out the process. There may also be a less conscious desire to confirm that a decision to withdraw treatment was, in fact, proper, and a quick death can validate such a decision. Physicians may encourage such thinking by stressing that the patient will certainly die soon without life-sustaining care and may mistakenly suggest that death will inevitably follow discontinuation in a very tidy manner, when in fact this does not always happen. Family members who have been following a patient during an acute illness are usually already exhausted when such a decision is made and out of their own suffering and personal time constraints may wish, consciously or unconsciously, for death to come sooner rather than later. Such feelings may prompt intense guilt in the bereaved. Finally, some patients and families deal with their living and dying like an on–off light switch. If they cannot have it all, they want it over as soon as possible. Physicians who do not understand this may be surprised when a patient or family that yesterday was asking for maximally aggressive care is today asking for a hastened death.

Prognosis, Palliative Care, and Hospice Eligibility

Prognosis is only one factor that needs to be considered in determining whether a patient would benefit from palliative or hospice care. Other factors to be considered are whether the system of care would best meet the patient's and family's needs and whether such care is in keeping with patient and family goals of care. Unfortunately, in the United States, influenced heavily by the Medicare Hospice Benefit, excessive weight has been given to life expectancy as a criterion for hospice eligibility. As originally formulated in the benefit, a patient is considered appropriate for hospice if he or she has a life expectancy of six months or less if the disease follows its natural course. As the discussion above reflects, this is easier to determine for some diseases, such as cancer, than for others.

Guidelines have been developed to help determine when hospice might be appropriate for patients with diseases other than cancer (and, by extension, when palliative care should also be considered). The evidence base for many of these guidelines is weak in terms of prognostic accuracy. Perhaps more important, the guidelines do not challenge more basic assumptions regarding the importance of prognosis in determining who might benefit from palliative or hospice care. For example, patients with dementia must be bedridden and virtually mute before hospice is considered "appropriate" in the United States. Speaking for myself, I will be ready for a hospice–palliative approach to care, stressing attention to quality of life and avoidance of acute care hospitals, long before I reach this level of debilitation. Patients sick enough to meet the criteria listed below are very sick indeed. They would likely benefit from consideration of palliative and hospice care in whatever form it is available.

Congestive Heart Failure: Class IV failure. Ejection fraction < 20%. Optimally treated, including afterload reduction. Two to three acute care admits for heart failure in the past year.

COPD: Oxygen dependent. Unresponsive to bronchodilators. Forced expiratory volume (FEV1) after bronchodilator less than 30% of predicted. At best able to walk only a few steps without tiring. Resting $pCO_2 > 50$, O_2 Sat off $O_2 < 88$, $pO_2 < 55$ on oxygen. Cor pulmonale, unintended weight loss > 10% of body weight, resting tachycardia > 100, two to three acute care admits for COPD in the past year.

Renal failure: Chronic renal failure with creatinine > 8.0, off dialysis.

Cirrhosis/liver failure: Spends most of time in bed, albumin < 2.5, INR > 1.5. At least one of the following co-morbidities: encephalopathy history of spontaneous bacterial peritonitis, refractory ascites, recurrent variceal bleeding, hepatorenal syndrome.

Dementia: Largely mute, bed-bound, unable to ambulate without assistance. History of recurrent aspiration pneumonias. Progressive weight loss. At or beyond stage seven of the Functional Assessment Staging scale. Urinary and fecal incontinence. Presence of co-morbid conditions in the past year: aspiration pneumonia, pyelonephritis, sepsis, decubitus ulcers, fever after antibiotics, difficulty swallowing or eating food, unintended weight loss of >10% over last six months.

Strokes/coma: *Acute phase*: Coma or persistent vegetative state secondary to stroke beyond three day's duration. Coma with any four of the following on day three of coma: abnormal brain stem response, absent verbal response, absent withdrawal response to pain, serum creatinine > 1.5, age >70. Dysphagia severe enough to prevent a patient from receiving food and fluids who declines or is not a candidate for artificial nutrition and hydration.

Chronic phase: Clear-cut predictors have not been as well classified. Consider the following: poor functional status with Karnofsky score <50%, post-stroke dementia with Functional Assessment Staging System (FAST) score > 7, poor nutritional status whether on artifical nutrition or not, > 10% weight loss over past six months, serum albumin < 2.5. Recurrent medical complications such as aspiration pneumonia, pyelonephritis, sepsis, refractory stage three to four decubiti, recurrent fever following antibiotics.

(Adapted from *Medical Guidelines for Determining Prognosis in Selected Non-Cancer Diseases*, 2nd ed. National Hospice Organization, Arlington Va., 1996.)

The Fantasy Death

So far, we have been talking in generalities. Let us bring things a little closer to home. How do you want to die? The question is not whether you wish to die, but given that you have no choice in the matter, what would be your preference? In working with physicians-in-training I often start with this question. I ask them to consider the most wonderful death they can imagine for themselves and then describe it, like a scene in a play. Many are taken aback and have trouble answering. Some answer immediately, as if they have been just waiting for someone to ask. I have heard a wide variety of responses. Nevertheless, I am struck by some persistent themes. They suggest common hopes and fears about dying.

Often the first respondent imagines dying suddenly, usually while asleep. An interesting variation on this theme was a newly married woman who hoped to die instantly and unknowingly with her husband in a plane explosion on the way back from a wonderful vacation to Hawaii. These sudden-death fantasies highlight a fear shared by many of us that dying will be painful and difficult. The best one can hope for is simply to disappear. As Woody Allen put it, "It's not that I'm afraid to die . . . I just don't want to be there when it happens." When such a sudden-death fantasy first appears, there is usually embarrassed laughter in sympathy by others in the group. Often someone mentions that what might be seen as "winning the game" by the dying individual would be viewed as the greatest of tragedies by family and friends. (The newlywed in her fantasy tried to trump this concern by dying simultaneously with her husband). Couples in a common spousal game may even discuss who "wins" based on who dies first. Often the first to die is seen as the winner, as the bereaved is left to mourn.

The second-most-common fantasy death takes place at home. Typically, participants describe a peaceful scene. In advanced but previously healthy old age, the dying person lies on the deathbed surrounded by family and friends. The home may be a literal home, a summer get-away cottage, or a fantasy home. In this fantasy people usually say they know they are dying. I will often ask, "How much time do you want to know you are dying?" Responses vary, but two weeks is common. The challenge in this question is that respondents are struggling between a sense that there is something to accomplish in dying (at least goodbyes to be said) and the fact that dying is still a scary business. Even in fantasy deaths, in which everybody is always physically comfortable, simply knowing you are to die soon is stressful. In fact, patients who get only two weeks notice usually perceive and are perceived as having virtually no time to come to grips with dying.

The third-most-common fantasy is dying while engaged in a valued or meaningful activity, often in a beautiful natural setting. A golfer wanted to die after a hole-in-one on the 18th hole. A mountain climber actually wanted to die with a rope breaking. A revolutionary wanted to die in a revolutionary struggle. Often, people describe pastoral scenes, dying on a mountaintop or drifting out to sea during a spectacular sunset.* One fantasy that combined a personal interest with nature and family had the dying person enjoying a party with loved ones on a glacier on a clear, cold night. The person then skis down the glacier off a cliff and flies out over the ocean, where he conveniently disappears.

It is remarkable how difficult it is for people really to see themselves in their death scenes. What is described is the scene, not the dying person. The dying person often seems to have been cut out from the scene. I suspect this reflects an understandable resistance to imagining oneself as old or actually dying.

Other than the sudden death fantasy, all fantasies I have heard seem to reflect, first and foremost, a sense of being at home. This home is often literal but may be figurative. A self-defined revolutionary is most at home in a revolution. This home seems to be even more important than comfort per se. No fantasy I have heard has included any discomfort. Even the revolutionary wanted to die

---

*Feifel in the 1950's found exactly the same rank ordering of preferences for types of death—sudden death, death at home, and what he described as "personal idiosyncrasies"—death "in a garden," "overlooking the ocean," "in a hammock on a spring day."[22] Aries points out that this fantasy favoring sudden death contrasts sharply with a more ancient belief that viewed sudden death as suspicious. "A sudden death was a vile and ugly death; it was frightening; it seemed a strange and monstrous thing that nobody dared talk about."[23]

"with a good clean head-shot." When even very young doctors describe this home, they often get goofy half-smiles on their faces and become surprisingly peaceful.

I have come to believe that finding one's home at the end of life is the central aspiration of dying people, understandable even to young physicians who are hopefully far from death. Helping people *connect* with their homes is our principle goal. Enhancing comfort is *not* the goal of hospice or palliative care but a means by which we remove obstacles to such connection. It is a very rare person who can be at home while in immense pain or while vomiting. While enhancing comfort and relieving suffering is a central *task* in providing hospice care, this is not adequate in and of itself. Helping people connect to their homes is truly the art of hospice and must draw upon the efforts of many who support the dying person.

For those who work with the dying, a critically related question is "How can we be at home in the face of the great suffering we are called to witness?" Dying people are remarkably sensitive to the emotional states of people around them. Our anxieties and fears are highly contagious. Mercifully, so, too, is peace and love. Such a question may seem overwhelming to a young doctor but can be easily understood if one imagines what one would like to see in one's own doctor in a crisis. Imagine having been in a car accident and then being wheeled into an emergency room. You need a chest tube (a very unpleasant procedure in which a large plastic tube is inserted between your ribs). A doctor approaches you. What do you want to see? You do *not* want to see that physician reading the instruction manual on how to insert chest tubes. Lack of experience and competence is not reassuring in the ER or in palliative care. Do you want to see someone who empathizes so much with your situation that he or she vomits or faints? I doubt it. Do you want a hardened, anesthetized physician who simply says, "Little stick" before jamming a tube into your chest? Certainly not. You want a physician who is competent and who can relate to your pain yet seems to radiate confidence and tranquility. It is no different in palliative care. However, really learning how to do this is so difficult that it is a lifetime practice. Personally, I am far, far from mastery.

Finally, it is remarkable what is not included in the fantasies. No fantasy has included a hospital, a physician, or a nurse. This should be humbling for those of us who work with the dying. We are *not* part of their fantasy—we are there because, sadly, most deaths are not ideal. People need help, and we are fortunate enough to be in a position to provide it.

References

1. Christakis, N. A. *Death Foretold: Prophecy and Prognosis in Medical Care.* 1999, University of Chicago Press: Chicago.

2. Becker, G. *Disrupted Lives—How People Create Meaning in a Chaotic World*. 1999, University of California Press: Berkeley.
3. Frank, A. *The Wounded Storyteller—Body, Illness, and Ethics*. 1995, University of Chicago Press: Chicago.
4. Knaus, W. et al. APACHE II: A severity of disease classification. Crit Care Med 1985; 13: 818–29.
5. Kosko, B. *Fuzzy Thinking—The New Science of Fuzzy Logic*. 1993, Hyperion: New York.
6. Forster, L. E. and J. Lynn. Predicting life span for applicants to inpatient hospice. Arch Intern Med 1988; 148(12): 2540–3.
7. Christakis, N. A. and J. J. Escarce. Survival of Medicare patients after enrollment in hospice programs. N Engl J Med 1996; 335(3): 172–8.
8. Viganò, A. et al. The relative accuracy of the clinical estimation of the duration of life for patients with end of life cancer. Cancer 1999; 86(1): 170–6.
9. Fisher, G., J. Tulsky, et al. Communicating a poor prognosis. In: R. Portenoy and E. Bruera, eds. *Topics in Palliative Care*. 2000, Oxford University Press: New York, pp. 75–91.
10. Gustafson, E. Dying: The career of the nursing home patient. J Health Soc Behav 1972; 13: 226–35.
11. Shneidman, E. *Deaths of Man*. 1973, Quadrangle: New York.
12. SUPPORT. A controlled trial to improve care for seriously ill hospitalized patients. The Study to Understand Prognoses and Preferences for Outcomes and Risks of Treatments (SUPPORT). JAMA 1995; 274(20): 1591–8.
13. Glaser, B. G. and A. L. Strauss. *Awareness of Dying*. 1965, Aldine: Chicago.
14. Teno, J. M. et al. Dying trajectory in the last year of life: Does cancer trajectory fit other diseases? Journal of Palliative Medicine 2001; 4(4): 457–64.
15. Lynn, J. and A.M. Wilkinson. Quality end of life care: The case for a MediCaring demonstration. Hospice Journal 1998; 13(1–2): 151–63.
16. Claessens, M. T. et al. Dying with lung cancer or chronic obstructive pulmonary disease: Insights from SUPPORT. Study to Understand Prognoses and Preferences for Outcomes and Risks of Treatments. J Am Geriatr Soc 2000; 48(5 suppl): S146–53.
17. Fox, E. et al. Evaluation of prognostic criteria for determining hospice eligibility in patients with advanced lung, heart, or liver disease. SUPPORT Investigators. Study to Understand Prognoses and Preferences for Outcomes and Risks of Treatments. JAMA 1999; 282(17): 1638–45.
18. Levenson, J. W. et al. The last six months of life for patients with congestive heart failure. J Am Geriatr Soc 2000; 48(5 suppl): S101–9.
19. Lynn, J. Caring at the end of our lives. New Engl J Med 1996; 335: 201–2.
20. Curtis, J. and G. D. Rubenfeld, eds. *Managing Death in the Intensive Care Unit*. 2001, Oxford University Press: New York.
21. Faber-Langendoen, K. and P. N. Lanken. Dying patients in the intensive care unit: Forgoing treatment, maintaining care. Ann Intern Med 2000; 133(11): 886–93.
22. Feifel, H. Attitudes toward death in some normal and mentally ill populations. In: H. Feifel, ed. *The Meaning of Death*. 1959, McGraw-Hill: New York, pp. 114–30.
23. Aries, P. *The Hour of Our Death*. 1981, Knopf: New York.

3

Symptom Management—Overview

Here am I, dying of a hundred good symptoms.

Alexander Pope

There are two paths to progress; one may enter through the path of **principle** or one may enter through the path of **technique**. Principle and technique are firmly tied together. At the very heart of every technique lies a basic principle. Look beyond technique and discover the principle. That gives it life. Technique is the hammer that drives the principle into our consciousness. Without technique—the principle has no way to express itself—it is just an idea.

Yagyu Jubei, Japanese swordsman

When I first met Mr. M. he was curled up in bed in a darkened room, looking resigned to his fate. I had read his chart and heard a short story explaining why he had been admitted to the nursing home.

"Mr. M. is an 86-year-old white male with rheumatoid arthritis, who has been living alone with his wife at home. His functional status has been gradually declining over the past few months to the extent that he can no longer transfer solo from bed to wheelchair. His wife has been helping, but she too is frail and cannot handle him any more. He is here for long-term placement."

29

From Mr. M. I heard a somewhat different story. Indeed, he had had rheumatoid arthritis for many years. It was now "burned-out"—the fires of redness and swelling had passed, leaving in their wake gnarled hands and other joints useless for even simple tasks such as buttoning his shirt, and, yes, he had been loosing ground. He had become "frozen," unable to move most all of his joints. His wife tried to help, but he was worried about her health. Rather than drag her down, too, he thought it better to come to the nursing home where, he assumed, he would die in the not distant future—or so he hoped.

He had pain, lots of pain, eight of ten on a pain scale, although this did not do justice to his experience. His pain had become inseparable from his frozen state. I asked what he had done, what he had taken for his pain. He had tried to keep his joints as flexible as he could, but it just hurt too much to move them. The pain of movement was replaced by a different pain of immobility—damned if he did and damned if he did not. He was still taking monthly gold injections for his arthritis, but these did not help his pain. He had taken naproxen, which had helped his pain significantly, but the doctors had stopped that a little over a year earlier, when he had had an episode of upper intestinal bleeding. He had tried Tylenol with codeine; it did not help much, and the constipation was as bad as the pain.

I reviewed his chart again, including numerous clinic notes. Pain was mentioned only in passing. Nonsteroidals (NSAIDs) were "contraindicated" because of the gastrointestinal bleeding. The patient had refused Tylenol with codeine. There was nothing more to do.

After thinking a bit, I talked with the patient again. I told him I would like to try some different therapies that might help him with his pain, and, perhaps, we could get his joints moving better. I could make no promises, but we would try. That was OK with him. I thought he would benefit from a low dose of a long-acting opioid, this time given with senna to counteract the constipation. I also wanted to rethink the NSAID issue. (This was before the availability of safer COX2 inhibitors.) I said, "You told me the naproxen helped your pain in the past. It's true that you are at a higher risk of bleeding again than most people. I can give you some additional medicine that should decrease the risk of your bleeding again to approximately 5–10% over the next year, but it is still a real risk. Are you willing to take this risk?" I will never forget it. He uncurled a bit and gave me an angry, penetrating glare. "Here I am, a bunch of pain just waiting to die. I'm 85, separated from the woman I love because I can't get around. You think I give a damn about a 10% chance of bleeding or dying? GIVE ME THE GODDAMN NAPROXEN!"

And so I did. We also used the opioid and briefly a TENS (transcutaneous electrical nerve stimulation) unit. We dipped his hands in paraffin. His pain decreased significantly. He began to loosen up. With physical therapy he regained his ability to transfer from bed to wheelchair on his own, and with this was able to return home to live with his wife.

The care I provided for Mr. M. was nothing special. He required no fancy pain control tricks. What was unusual about this case? I had brought Mr. M. into the decision-making process, allowing him to weigh the risk of bleeding again against potential pain relief. Why had not his former physicians? One reason, I think, is that his physicians had come to worry more about the harm that might be done than the good that might be accomplished. Probably for his physicians, gastrointestinal bleeding loomed large as a life-threatening complication, which it can be. However, *pain*—that was something else, hard to measure, an intangible symptom. From the physicians' perspective the trade-off was great enough that the possibility of continuing naproxen simply was not on the "menu;" there was no choice to offer. NSAIDS were "contraindicated."

In medical school and residency training I learned very little about symptom management. For the most part I learned by imitation. A resident one month used this suppository for nausea, so I did too. The next month another resident used a different suppository and that, too, was OK. After all, one size fits all, I thought, but I was wrong. I was amazed in my early palliative care training to learn how much antiemetics differed in their actions. As I came to understand how much could be done for patients to help them feel better, I wondered why I had not been taught this before.

The *New Oxford Dictionary* provides the following definition of a symptom: "A physical or mental phenomenon, circumstance or change of condition arising from and accompanying a disorder and constituting evidence for it . . . specifically a subjective indicator perceptible to the patient and as opposed to an objective one (compare with sign)."[1] A symptom represents a *clue* to something more important. We often say, "That's only a symptom. The real problem is. . . ." In our system of medicine the real problem is the *disease*. This choice of wording, this understanding, is unfortunate, as it devalues symptoms. Clues are interesting as long as the mystery remains unsolved. However, once solved, clues are soon forgotten. For most patients who could benefit from palliative care, the mystery, the disease, has long since been revealed. Perhaps this is one reason modern clinicians have so roundly ignored symptom management as a proper focus of medicine.

The perspective of patients is quite different. Patients do not so much have symptoms as *experiences* of illness.[2] Mr. M., suffering with the pain of rheumatoid arthritis, would have found it ludicrous to consider his pain merely a clue to "something more important." Experientially, symptoms are inseparable from the disease. Pain is part of rheumatoid arthritis. Classic symptoms are still important in providing clues to as yet undiscovered disease processes. If we can identify a previously unknown disease, our efforts to treat the experience of illness will usually be much enhanced. However, when considering symptom management of known, chronic illnesses, what is usually more important is to understand what clues the *disease* process can provide us to understand and treat the symptoms, the experiences, of the patient. Understanding the nature of pain in rheumatoid arthritis aided us in devising a strategy that helped Mr. M. with his experience. Thus, in palliative care we often reverse the relationship between the disease and the symptom; the disease process becomes a clue to the symptom/experience.

Palliative Case Note

Ask the question—what does the *disease* process tell us about the patient's *symptoms.*

Most symptoms have physical and psychic components. The physical pathophysiologic component can further be subdivided into *local* and *central* physiologies. For example, Mr. M.'s pain arose both from local processes in his joints and central processes that register pain. Optimal management requires understanding both these central and local physiologies. The following chapters on such common symptoms as pain and nausea will emphasize understanding and addressing these local and central physiologies. However, in the care of the individual patient, the totality of physical and psychic aspects of the experience must be addressed.

The psychic component of symptoms can be subdivided into affective (emotional), cognitive, and spiritual components, which are closely intertwined and integrated with the physical experience of illness. Optimal management requires some understanding of how these psychic components are integrated into the experience and adjusting care accordingly. A pain that is primarily spiritual in nature, for example, will not respond well to morphine but may respond to spiritual counseling (Fig. 3.1).

Affective Components of Symptom Management

How do we *feel* when ill—depressed, angry, scared, panicky, anxious, embarrassed, threatened, guilty, exhausted, hopeless, or sad? Affect comes in many colors. It is often tightly linked to physical experience. Mr. M.'s pain had shades of depression, resignation, and anger. Severe dyspnea associated with air-hunger, for example, can induce pure panic. Our emotional states are also greatly affected by cognitive processes. The *meaning* of an illness affects how we emotionally experience that illness. Dyspnea associated with jogging, for example, may mean that the person has just had a good workout and actually is enjoying life. A similar physical stimulus to a patient dying of lung cancer may mean impending death. A myriad of emotions may follow that become part of the experience of dyspnea—anger or guilt about smoking, sadness, and panic, for example. Depression, anxiety, and grief will be explored in greater depth in chapter 7.

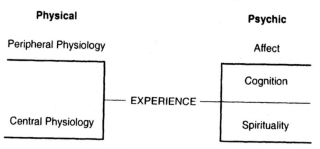

Figure 3.1. The experience of illness.

Cognitive Components of Symptom Management

The cognitive component of symptoms refers to the organization of the experience into a framework that is intelligible and meaningful. Cognition is not necessarily rational. A delirious patient who complains about being stabbed by devils may have an underlying physical cause for pain, such as a broken rib or other lesion. This may be interpreted cognitively as being a devil, with the affective response being terror. Cognition allows organization of a complex experience into something like a story, thus making the experience intelligible. The story has meaning: "Being stabbed by a devil means I'm in serious trouble." Thus, in trying to interpret the cognitive component, attention should be paid both to organizational *structure* and its implied *meaning* and associated affect. The organization and meaning of the experience will be shaped by previous personal and cultural experiences and beliefs as well as the mental capacity and orientation of the patient. The same delirious patient who experiences pain as a devil may have normal intelligence, but the experience is affected not only by earlier experience, such as a belief in devils, but by the patient's altered mental status.

I could never fully understand how Mr. M. experienced his pain. Clearly, more than simple physical discomfort was involved. His joint pains were interwoven with a more total pain of his experience.[3,4] Pain meant more than "ouch." I imagine for Mr. M. pain meant many things—being frozen, helpless, dependent, isolated, and separated from people and things he loved, among others. Analyzing the cognitive component requires understanding both the patient's story and organization of the experience and implied meanings.

Spiritual Components of Symptom Management

Not all symptoms are experienced with spiritual or religious overtones. It is quite possible to be constipated or scratch an itch without pondering deeper meanings. However, spirituality often plays a major role in the experience of illness, and certain symptoms simply cannot be comprehended or addressed without considering spirituality. For some the importance of religion or spirituality is obvious. "Was this illness inflicted by God or a devil? Is this a curse?" they may ask. For many, deeper levels of meaning can be considered spiritual without being overtly religious. Suffering calls upon us to make sense of our pain, to integrate our experience with our view of what makes the universe tick, and then decide how we should respond—prayer, resignation, a fighting spirit, or perhaps a quest? If we as clinicians are to make any sense of our patients' experiences, we will do so only if we get some notion of how their experiences fit into their larger life stories, which, ultimately, revolve around deeply rooted meanings and values.

So, what symptoms are we talking about? In thumbing through the index of the *Oxford Textbook of Palliative Medicine*, I identified 54 different symptoms: constipation, diarrhea, peripheral edema, nausea/vomiting, pruritus/itching, dyspnea, anxiety, anorexia, sleep disorders, cough, akathisia, dysphagia, anhedonia, death rattle/secretions, depression, drooling, urinary incontinence, rectal incontinence, hiccups, flatulence, muscle spasms, confusion, memory loss, visual problems, hearing loss, dysgeusia, colic, sexual dysfunction, polyuria, polydipsia, dizziness, dyspepsia, xerostomia, dry skin, dysarthria, dysphoria, dysuria, failure to thrive, fatigue, fear, fever, hallucinations, halitosis, impotence, irritability, taste alterations, odor, mucositis, pain, panic attacks, photosensitivity, restlessness, stomatitis, and urinary frequency. (I may have missed some, and others might get different numbers depending on whether they are lumpers or splitters.) It would be impossible to cover them all in this text. However, I hope to illustrate specific points in symptom management by addressing certain common symptoms. Little explanation is needed for the inclusion of pain, the archetypical symptom and experience of suffering. A discussion of nausea and vomiting reveals the extent to which our understanding of basic pathophysiology at a receptor level has enabled us to tailor symptom management to specific receptor mechanisms. Dyspnea illustrates, perhaps better than any other symptom, the totality of experience in body, mind, and spirit that gives rise to suffering. Mouth and bowel care are unglamorous aspects of care, often overlooked by physicians, but are absolutely essential for quality of life. The discussion of bowel obstruction highlights the need for further research to link an understanding of physiology with treatment. The medical treatment of bowel obstruction is also incredibly challenging, technically. If any problem other than pain were to be the "poster child" for why we need some specialists in palliative care, it would be bowel obstruction.

References

1. Doyle, D., G. W. C. Hanks, et al. *Oxford Textbook of Palliative Medicine*, 2nd ed. 1998, Oxford University Press: New York, p. 203.

2 Hahn, R. *Sickness and Healing—An Anthropological perspective*. 1995, Yale University Press: New London, Conn., pp. 1–56.

3. Saunders, C. M. The philosophy of terminal care. In: C. M. Saunders, ed. *The Management of Terminal Disease*. 1978, Arnold: London, pp. 193–202.

4. Clark, D. "Total pain," disciplinary power and the body in the work of Cicely Saunders, 1958–1967. Soc Sci Med 1999; 49(6): 727–36.

4

Pain Management

Always the same. Now a spark of hope flashes up, then a sea of
despair rages, and always pain; always pain, and always the same.
                          Leo Tolstoy, *The Death of Ivan Ilych*

All of us experience pain in life. People look to clinicians for relief from pain
when it becomes difficult to bear. Our duty to alleviate the suffering engendered
by pain harkens back to the very roots of what it means to be a healer. Recent
advances in the understanding and treatment of pain allow us to fulfill this ob-
ligation to our patients far better than we ever could before. Unfortunately, new
pain relief methods are too often underused or poorly used.

Pain is the most common presenting complaint to physicians in North America,
and I suspect this is true in other regions of the world.[1] It has been estimated
that 85% to 95% of pain syndromes, including severe forms, such as cancer-
related pain, can be adequately palliated using relatively simple techniques.[2]
However, pain is often under-treated. In one study of cancer patients at a
famous cancer center, as many as 50% of cancer patients suffered unrelieved
pain.[3] Such under-treatment of pain is not isolated to cancer. The SUPPORT
study demonstrated that 50% of the 9105 patients studied were estimated by
surviving relatives as having moderate or severe pain 50% of the time or more
in the last three days of life.[4] A study of the treatment of nonmalignant pain in

49,971 nursing home patients found that 25% of patients with daily pain received no analgesics whatsoever. Advanced age (>85), male sex, cognitive impairment, and being a member of a racial minority were statistically significant risk factors for receiving no analgesics.[5]

Classification of Pain

Acute Pain

We all have experienced acute pain. Bee stings, bumped knees, and bone fractures are simple examples. Most acute pain serves a clear purpose: some problem needs to be addressed. Acute pain is characterized by help-seeking behavior. In most cases people cry out and move about in a very obvious manner. Physiologic responses to acute pain include tachycardia, tachypnea, and sweating due to discharge in the sympathetic nervous system. It is easy to recognize and empathize with acute pain. It is practically automatic. We wince if we see severe, acute pain and respond with our own "sympathetic" discharge.

The treatment of acute pain can be difficult in that the intensity of pain may change dramatically over a short period of time. Physicians may have trouble adjusting pain medications rapidly enough to match the level of pain being experienced because pain intensity tends to escalate and decrease swiftly. Both under- and overtreatment can easily occur. Undertreatment risks excessive suffering. Overtreatment poses real medical risks. Thus, as acute pain changes rapidly, treatment of such pain requires frequent reassessment of the patient's status in order to avoid extremes of under- and overtreatment.

Chronic Pain

Chronic pain is very different from acute pain. It serves no biological purpose. While the suffering engendered may be as great as is that in acute pain, it is subjectively experienced and objectively displayed in a very different way. For reasons not well understood, chronic pain is characterized by physical and mental withdrawal. Vegetative signs very similar to those found in depression, such as anorexia, anhedonia, lethargy, and sleep disturbance are often present. Chronic pain frequently coexists with depression, making it difficult at times to distinguish between the two. Obvious displays of distress, as are found in acute pain, are usually absent. Chronic pain is very difficult to recognize. Even when recognized we tend not to experience the same intense, visceral empathy that arises so easily in the presence of acute pain. Lack of recognition of chronic pain and difficulty empathizing with it are major barriers to successful treatment.

It is difficult to judge by observation alone the degree of chronic pain suffered. Both family members and professional health care workers tend to miss the mark. Tragically, the correlation between a patient's and another's assessment of pain intensity is poorer at higher degrees of pain. In one study using visual analog scales (VAS) from 0 to 10 to measure pain intensity, correlation between the observers' estimated intensity score and that reported by the patient was worst at high levels of pain, scores of 7 to 10 (severe to unendurable).[6] This stands in dramatic contrast to our experience with acute pain; the more severe the acute pain the easier it is for us to recognize. From this and other studies it has been concluded that for patients with chronic pain, we cannot simply "see" if a patient is in pain. We are, in effect, "color-blind" to chronic pain. We also cannot judge the degree of pain by measures such as noting how calm or disturbed a patient appears. In a manner of speaking we suffer a disability. As with any disability, we must try to find ways to compensate. In order to determine how much pain a patient is in, we have to *ask*. If possible, it is advisable to use a scale of pain intensity to communicate intensity of pain. Numeric scales from 0 to 5 or 0 to 10 or visual analogue scales, some with pictures reflecting varying degrees of distress, are commonly used. These allow a better assessment of pain intensity and a more accurate measure of changes with therapeutic intervention.

Is it reasonable or necessary to measure pain on a routine basis? I would argue that the evidence is overwhelming that people simply lack the proper receptors to detect chronic pain (much like we cannot *see* blood pressure). It would be wonderful if all clinicians routinely asked patients about their pain. However, the evidence is also strong that clinicians have resisted efforts to improve pain assessment less formally. However, is such measurement scientific?

Pain management would be infinitely easier if we had something like an O_2 saturation meter to measure pain—something like the tricorder in Star Trek movies. Clinicians prefer hard data and become uncomfortable with subjective reports. In an absolute sense we cannot know if one patient's 7 to 10 pain is the same as that of another. However, studies have demonstrated that the individual patient is consistent in reporting pain scores. That is, intra-rater reliability has been validated.[7] I think of pain scores as imperfect tools to compensate for our collective disability.

Even so, what if people lie? In hospice literature it has been said that pain is whatever the patient says it is. This seems a bit simplistic to me. While it is true that we are color-blind to chronic pain, it is also true that some patients may be less than honest about their pain. Patients may fabricate or exaggerate symptoms for psychological reasons or secondary gain. Patients with very real chronic pain may also learn to exaggerate their pain and become demanding, as they believe physicians will not otherwise take them seriously, a process called "pseudo-addiction."[8] Paradoxically, this may arouse suspicion in the practitioner that the pain is not "real." There is no easy way to tell what is real. However, common sense and a trusting relationship between provider and patient go a long way. As a general rule, if the complaint of pain is plausible and if there are no very good reasons for doubting the patient, believe it. My philosophy is that ties go to the patient. Of two possible "sins" in pain management, the sin of ignoring real pain seems greater than does the sin of occasionally being fooled by a patient.

Palliative Care Note

When not sure whether the patient is telling the truth or not about pain, ties go to the patient.

Types of Pain

There are two major types of pain, nociceptive and neuropathic. Distinguishing between them is important because the causes and treatments are different. Ideally, the causes of both types of pain will be identified and treated, resulting in pain relief. Unfortunately, it is often the case that cure is impossible and palliation is necessary.

Nociceptive (Tissue) Pain

Nociceptive pain results from tissue damage. Intact neurons dutifully report damage, and pain is experienced. Nociceptive pain can be subdivided into somatic and visceral (gut) pain. Nociceptive pain can be experienced as sharp, dull, or aching. There may be radiation of the pain, especially visceral pain, but it will *not* be in a direct nerve distribution. For example, gallbladder pain can radiate to the scapula. Nociceptive pain is generally responsive to NSAIDs (nonsteroidal anti-inflammatory drugs) and opioids. Conditions associated with inflammation, bone pain, and joint disease are particularly responsive to NSAIDs.

Neuropathic (Nerve) Pain

Neuropathic pain may occur when there is either damage to or dysfunction of nerves in the peripheral or central nervous system. Faulty signals are sent to the brain and experienced as pain. Neuropathic pain can be either peripheral (outside the central nervous system) or central in origin. Examples of neuropathic pain include diabetic neuropathy, trigeminal neuralgia, postherpetic zoster pain (peripheral pains), and the thalamic pain syndrome (a central pain). Neuropathic pain frequently coexists with nociceptive pain. Examples include trauma that damages tissue and nerves, burns (that burn skin as well as nerve endings), and external nerve compression. Examples of the latter include tumor nerve compression and sciatica from herniated discs pressing on nerves.

Neuropathic pain is often described as having a burning or electrical quality. It may feel like a shock or lightning bolt. Sometimes stimuli that usually do not cause pain, such as light touch, may elicit a paroxysm of pain. A light stroke of the cheek that results in the sudden pain of trigeminal neuralgia is an example of this type of pain. Sometimes patients do not describe the sensation as being "painful" but rather as feeling unpleasantly strange or tingly, like an arm feels when it wakes up from "going to sleep." This is called a dysesthesia. Diabetic neuropathy commonly results in this type of sensation.

Neuropathic pain in the peripheral nervous system frequently follows a nerve distribution. This distribution may replicate a particular nerve, as in sciatic pain or trigeminal neuralgia, or may represent the distribution of terminal nerve endings, as in the stocking-glove distribution of peripheral neuropathies.

Neuropathic pain is relatively resistant to NSAIDs and opioids, although they may be helpful in certain cases. The other major classes of medications useful for neuropathic pain, tricyclic antidepressants, anticonvulsants, and sodium channel blockers, will be discussed later.

Evaluation of Pain

As discussed earlier, pain is a complex and personal experience. It is affected by physiological, psychological, and spiritual factors. The evaluation of pain must consider these factors and their interactions that result in the experience of pain. A useful mnemonic in evaluating pain(s) is the acronym: NOPQRST.[9]

N: Number of Pains
Although we tend to speak of a patient's pain as an overall experience, in fact, many patients have more than one pain. It would be more appropriate to speak of a patient's *pains*. These should be individually evaluated.

O: Origin of Pain
Understanding the cause of a particular pain is immensely helpful. Removal of the underlying cause may eliminate the pain. Even if this is not possible, understanding the origin of the pain may help with consideration of specific therapeutic options.

P: Palliate and Potentiate
What makes the pain better or worse? Do certain activities or body positions alleviate or worsen the pain? How have previously tried medications affected the pain (partial relief, no relief, etc.)? This may provide an important clue as to the type of pain being experienced, if in doubt. While the focus of this text is on pharmacologic therapy, it is important to point

out that nonpharmacologic interventions can have a significant (positive or negative) effect on pain.

Nociceptive pain tends to worsen when stress or pressure is applied to an affected area. Neuropathic pain may be "set off" when usually nonpainful stimuli, such as a light touch, temperature change, or even air movement, provoke a "reverb"-like phenomenon, with paroxysms of pain.

While patients may be able to speak about the effect of medications or body positions, they may be less able to comment on the effect of psychological or spiritual factors. The clinician should be aware that depression, anxiety, confusion, and spiritual distress may all contribute significantly to the experience of pain. If these conditions are present, treating them may result in significant palliation.

Q: Quality

A great variety of words are used to describe pain. Nociceptive pain may be sharp, dull, stabbing, or pressurelike. Neuropathic pain descriptions often have an electrical quality: burning, lancinating, buzzing, tingling, zapping, and lightninglike.

R: Radiation

Both nociceptive and neuropathic pains may radiate, although we usually associate radiation with neuropathic pain. Neuropathic pain tends to radiate in a distribution that follows nerves. Classic examples include trigeminal neuralgia and herpes zoster pain. The stocking glove distribution of peripheral neuropathies, as in diabetes, also follows a pattern of terminal nerve endings. Nociceptive pain radiates in less obvious ways. Thus, pericarditis, for example, may radiate to the scapula. Cardiac pain may radiate to the arm(s) or neck.

S: Severity/Suffering

Severity. As mentioned above, it is impossible to accurately gauge the severity of chronic pain by observation alone. You have to ask. The use of pain scales is strongly recommended when patients report having pain. Some patients respond better to certain scales than others. Some scales use nonnumerical images such as faces or colors to represent the range of distress.

Having said this, even numerical scales communicate limited data. On a scale of 0 to 10, is one person's 7 the same as another's? How many of us have really experienced level 10 pain? What is the worst pain we could endure? Hopefully, we will never find out.

If nothing else, pain scales seem to communicate the patient's urgency in wanting their pain addressed. On a scale of 0 to 10, pains of 1 to 3 are often well tolerated. Patients often decline additional interventions at these levels. Levels 3 to 6 usually indicate that some intervention is desired, although it is not an emergency. Pain at 7 to 10 is a serious problem. Not only is the pain seriously distressing, there is usually a fear that it will become a 10 and thus "out of control." Pain at level 10 (or greater) is perceived as an emergency by the patient and should usually be treated as an emergency by the clinician. Such pain is overwhelming. Having said this, some patients will report that pain management is "adequate" with a score as high as 7 to 10. Others will want urgent treatment when the scores rise from 1 to 2.6. Understanding how that patient interprets the pain score is most important. It is strongly advised that the examiner assess whether a given score means treatment is adequate for the individual patient. Individual patients tend to be consistent over time.

Suffering. What impact is the pain having on the patient? The impact may be an internal experience, such as depression or a thought of suicide, or may directly affect the patient's functioning. Sleep disturbances, difficulty walking, inability to work, and impairment of the activities of daily living may all reflect the pain experience. As obvious as this may seem, I am struck by how often we forget to ask how pain (or other symptoms) affect a person's life. Perhaps it is because we assume that pain is simply awful—what more do we need to know? However, hearing how a person is *suffering* with pain (both the nitty-gritty—"I can't work"—and the deep issues—"I wonder why God did this to me") helps us understand and empathize with what the patient is going through. Personally, I have trouble relating to a number, but if a patient can begin talking to me about how life has changed for them, then I feel I can gain a small glimpse of their experience.

T: Timing and Trend

Timing. Pain is rarely the same at all times. Pain has a pattern over time. Later, I will explain how matching the patient's pain pattern with therapeutic interventions (pattern matching) enables one to maximize therapeutic efficacy and minimize side effects, especially when treating nociceptive pain. Acute pain comes on rapidly and usually dissipates rapidly. Most chronic pain has a base and occasional spikes of incident pain, which may be predictable or unpredictable. Both need to be addressed. For example, some men may experience predictable trigeminal neuralgia only when shaving. Bed-bound patients often experience pain predictably with turning or cleaning. Wounds may hurt during dressing changes.

Trend. Pain often has momentum. It is very difficult to get a handle on rapidly escalating pain. Therapy is harder and suffering appears to be greater when the trend is worsening. This is true both physiologically and psychologically. Physically, we now know that escalating pain can "rev-up" in the central nervous system, amplifying painful stimuli and resulting in stronger pain signals. Specific receptors in the spinal cord such as those for N-methyl-D-aspartate (NMDA) are involved in this process, and blockading such receptors can be useful in resistant pain syndromes. Psychologically, patients are very aware of their pain trend. If the pain is worsening, patients understandably project into the future that it will become worse and even unendurable. This projection itself contributes to the pain experience and may be communicated as a higher pain score. Likewise, if the trend is good, patients may be able to tolerate more physical pain at any given moment as they project into a more pleasant future. Pain is certainly experienced in the present but is understood in terms of the past and the future.

Perhaps a personal story will help illustrate this point. A few years ago while having a dental cavity filled, I tried to distract myself from the pain I was experiencing by asking myself, "On a scale of 0 to 10, how much pain do you have," as I had asked countless patients. "Hmm, perhaps a 3 or a 4," I thought. With each little whine of the drill I thought, "Only a few moments more, then it will be over." I was to raise my hand if I had too much pain, but I could bear it a bit longer. And then it was over. I wondered—what if that pain had gone on forever? What if I had known it would not only go on, but get worse and worse? My hand would have been up in a flash. The idea of that pain going on and getting worse would have been too much to bear.

Pain Management Strategy

Having assessed the patient's pain, a strategy for management should be developed. The discussion that follows emphasizes opioids because these are so commonly used in palliative care. However, this is not to suggest that opioids are more or less appropriate in any individual case. Sound clinical judgment must be used in selecting specific agents.

What Nonpharmacologic Approaches to Pain Should Be Adopted?

Although the emphasis here is on the pharmacology of pain management, the clinician should also consider other interventions in developing a strategy. How does the patient's psychological state affect his or her pain? Is the patient depressed, anxious, or confused? How does the patient relate to his or her pain? Some patients want all pain to be abolished. Others may want some pain to remain. (As one cancer patient put it, "If I didn't feel some pain, how would I know what that cancer is doing in there.") Some may see the pain as something to be conquered. Some may see it as something to be accepted. A thorough discussion of the psychological and spiritual aspects of pain is beyond the scope of this text. Often, assistance from others—psychologists, psychiatrists, social workers, and chaplains—will be necessary if proper care is to be delivered.

A variety of medical interventions other than medications may also be extremely useful. Radiation therapy and chemotherapy may help alleviate pain in patients with certain cancers. Nerve blocks, trigger-point injections, and (rarely) surgical approaches may also be useful. Physical therapy, occupational therapy, and massage therapy may help in certain cases. Experts in these areas should be consulted, as needed.

Principles in Choosing Medications

1. **Avoid specific toxicities.** In choosing among possible medications, an otherwise useful drug might be excessively toxic for a particular patient. A patient with thrombocytopenia, for example, would be a poor candidate for a traditional nonsteroidal anti-inflammatory drug (NSAID), because such drugs interfere with platelet aggregation.
2. **Look for "two-fers."** When possible, identify agents with additional effects that might be beneficial—two for the price of one. Anticonvulsants, for example, might be particularly useful in a patient with a seizure disorder who also had neuropathic pain. In contrast, one might choose a tricyclic antidepressant (TCA) for neuropathic pain in a depressed patient.
3. **Think about who will be administering the medicine.** A medication that requires injection might be very appropriate in a hospital or nursing home but difficult to administer at home. Competent patients administering their own medications may be better able to manage short-acting pain medications on an as-needed basis. In contrast, a demented patient with pain cared for in a nursing home or at home by family will probably receive inadequate analgesia when treated q4 h prn, as family and staff may not assess pain regularly (especially at night) and the patient may be unable to advocate for him- or herself. Long-acting preparations of both NSAIDs and opioids may be more appropriate in such a situation.
4. **Consider the drug delivery route of administration.** Possible routes of therapy include oral, enteral tube, percutaneous and parenteral intravenous (IV), intramuscular (IM), and subcutaneous (SC). (See later discussion of routes of delivery)
5. **Identify the patient's *pain pattern* and perform *pattern matching* with your therapy.**

Pattern Matching

Management of pain is optimized when therapy overlaps the patient's pattern of pain. This maximizes analgesia while minimizing side effects. In using opioids for therapy when pain increases, so should the drug dose. Similarly, when pain lessens, the drug dose should be decreased. Pain itself can counteract certain opioid side effects. In particular, sedation and respiratory depression are significantly blocked by pain. Thus, the goal in using opioids is to have pain signals and opioid signals neutralize each other.

Acute pain, with a pattern of rapid escalation and de-escalation, requires short-acting opioids and careful titration if pain is to be adequately managed and side effects avoided (Fig. 4.1).

Chronic pain typically has both a background "noise" of pain with intermittent spikes of incident, or breakthrough, pain. The general strategy for such pain is to use a long-acting agent to manage the background basal pain and short-acting opioid doses as needed for breakthrough pain (Fig. 4.2).

While these are common patterns, the patient's individual pain pattern should be considered. For example, a patient may complain of pain only at night. This pattern should generate a "differential diagnosis" that may lead to important changes in therapy. This pattern may reflect pain worsened by lying down. Perhaps the patient is unable to get needed pain medications at night, as he or she is dependent on others, family, or nursing staff who may be less responsive during this time. Maybe he or she is no longer distracted, as in the daytime, which increases an awareness of pain. Each of these underlying causes would require a different approach.

Let us review the classes of common analgesics before getting into a more in depth discussion of routes of therapy and dosing strategies for opioids (Fig. 4.3).

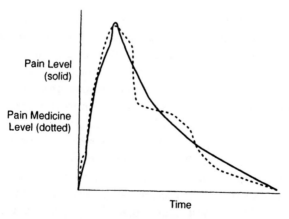

Time

Figure 4.1. Acute pain pattern matching. Analgesia is maximized and side effects minimized when the rise and fall of the blood level of an analgesic closely overlaps the temporal pattern of a patient's pain.

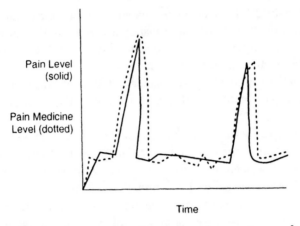

Pain Level (solid)

Pain Medicine Level (dotted)

Time

Figure 4.2. Chronic pain pattern. Generally, a long-acting medication for the baseline pain that is always present and a short-acting medication that rapidly peaks in tandem with an acute pain spike are needed.

Classes of Analgesics

Nonsteroidal Anti-Inflammatory Drugs (NSAIDs)

NSAIDs are a mainstay in the management of mild to moderate nociceptive pain. As mentioned above, they are particularly useful in inflammatory states and in pain involving the musculoskeletal system.[10] It is beyond the scope of this book to discuss the large number of NSAIDs available today. Rather, some guidelines for choosing and using them are offered.

1. Consider drug half-life and frequency of administration. Short-acting agents such as ibuprofen may be preferable for pain that arises intermittently and is of short duration. Such agents can be given on an as needed basis. For patients with chronic pain that requires round-the-clock analgesia, a longer-acting agent such as naproxen, which may allow more convenient dosing, may result in better patient compliance and improved analgesia.
2. It is a mistake to consider NSAIDs as necessarily less toxic than opioids. NSAIDs may cause upper intestinal symptoms such as heartburn, nausea, or vomiting in 10% to 20% of patients. Significant upper GI bleeding from either gastritis or duodenal ulceration can occur, as can nephrotoxicity. Bronchospasm may be precipitated in sensitive asthmatics, as with aspirin. NSAIDs can cause altered mental status, especially in the elderly and frail. Most NSAIDs inhibit platelet aggregation. This is particularly a risk in patients who receive anticoagulants and in patients with thrombocytopenia.

3. For some patients NSAIDs may be as effective or more effective than are opioids in relieving pain. In such cases it may be a mistake to withhold this class of medication for fear of some of these side effects. Rather, additional steps may be necessary to minimize the risk. Misoprostol, a prostaglandin E1 analog, can significantly reduce the risk of gastritis and gastric ulceration due to NSAIDs. Misoprostol is also effective against duodenal peptic ulceration. H2 blockers, such as ranitidine, have been found to reduce the risk of duodenal ulcers for patients treated with NSAIDs. Standard doses of H2 blockers such as famotidine 20 mg BID do not protect against NSAID-related gastric ulcers. However, one study with higher dose famotidine, 40 mg BID, did show a protective effect.[11] Identification and eradication of *H. pylori* infection may lessen the risk of bleeding with NSAIDs in those infected for both duodenal and gastric ulcers. When there is concern over renal function, careful monitoring of blood chemistries may allow early detection of adverse effects. If deterioration in renal function is detected, discontinuation of the NSAID usually results in a gradual return to baseline function. Use of COX2 inhibitors (see below) may also help minimize risk.

COX2 Inhibitors

Recently, a new class of NSAIDs has become available, the COX2 inhibitors.[12] Selective blockade of cyclooxygenase permits analgesia and an anti-inflammatory effect while minimizing the risk of GI toxicity and bleeding. Although experience in the use of these drugs in palliative care is limited, the following should be helpful in considering when to use one of these agents.

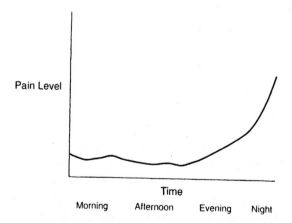

Figure 4.3. Pain exacerbation at night. What is the "differential diagnosis" for this kind of pain?

1. They are relatively expensive. This makes them considerably more expensive than naproxen, for example. However, in absolute terms, if an NSAID is truly indicated and significant contraindications exist for standard NSAIDs, the difference in price may be worth it.
2. They appear to be equi-efficacious with other NSAIDs but with no evidence of superior analgesia.
3. Evidence is strong that the risk of GI bleeding is significantly reduced with these agents.[13] When an NSAID is truly needed and there is concern about GI bleeding, the total cost may be lowered by using one of these agents rather than by adding a relatively expensive prophylactic drug such as misoprostol or a pump-inhibitor.
4. Evidence is strong that platelet aggregation is not inhibited by these agents. Thus, in patients with thrombocytopenia, defective platelets (uremia), and bleeding tendencies these drugs may offer a strong advantage.

Opioids—A Misunderstood Class of Drugs

Many misconceptions exist relative to the use of opioids. These misunderstandings have resulted in global underuse of these medications for pain relief. It is a mistake to extrapolate from the effects of opioids on addicts to the effects of opioids on patients in pain. Opioids used for pain relief act very differently on the body and mind than do opioids used by people not in pain. Most of the horrors observed in addicts do not occur in patients who take opioids for pain relief. The presence of pain itself changes the effect of opioids. When we administer opioids for pain relief, we do so considering the opioid to be an antidote to the poison of pain. Many are not aware that pain reciprocally acts, in part, as an antidote to certain of the toxic effects of opioids. Ideally, the effects of pain and opioids cancel each other out, allowing pain relief with minimal toxicity.

Palliative Care Note

Pain can serve as a partial antidote to certain opioid side effects—euphoria, sedation, and respiratory depression.

Pain also seems to block much of the euphoric effect of opioids. Contrary to popular thinking, the risk of turning a nonaddict into an addict when treating pain is very, very small to nonexistent. In one review by Porter, 11,882 patients without a prior history of addiction who were treated for pain with opioids were followed to determine how many developed addictive behavior. Only four did so.[14] A more recent study reviewed statistics on the medical use of opioids and the incidence of opioid abuse from 1990 to 1996 in the United States. It found that while medical use of opioids (except for meperidine) had increased dramatically over that period of time (morphine use up 59%), this trend was not paralleled by increased opioid abuse. It concluded, "The trend of increasing medical use of opioid analgesics to treat pain does not appear to contribute to increases in the health consequences of opioid analgesic abuse."[15] *Physical dependence* does occur with repeated dosing. However, such dependence does *not* result in craving for the drug, associated with deleterious life consequences (a definition of addiction). It is notable that many drugs cause similar dependence without addiction—meaning that sudden discontinuation of the drug results in adverse physiological effects. Beta blockers, clonidine, and steroids, among others, can result in physical dependence.

If pain is skillfully treated with opioids, adverse complications such as respiratory depression and significant sedation rarely occur. No good evidence base exists for the common belief that the proper use of opioids (compared to the use of opioids by addicts) in the treatment of pain hastens the chance of death. Mild sedation and nausea may occur with initiation of opioid therapy or with subsequent increases in dosing. These side effects relate more to increases in opioid dosing and serum levels than to the absolute amounts of opioid administered. They usually subside after steady state levels are achieved—usually in a day or two.

While sedation and nausea tend to resolve over time as steady serum levels are obtained, such is not the case with constipation. As a rule, patients receiving chronic opioid therapy require continuous laxative therapy. This need for laxatives should be anticipated at the outset of therapy and not when constipation becomes a problem, as it almost inevitably does. (See the section on constipation in Chapter 5.) Constipation is caused by opioids binding mu receptors in the intestinal tract. Patients on very high doses of opioids do not necessarily require higher laxative doses to compensate than do those on lower doses. Orally administered opioids may result in somewhat more severe constipation than does transdermally administered fentanyl, perhaps because of more concentrated mucosal exposure.[16,17]

Palliative Care Note

Side effects related primarily to rising serum opioid levels are sedation, nausea and vomiting, and respiratory depression. Effects related primarily to steady state opioid levels are pain and dyspnea relief and constipation.

Many physicians fail to prescribe opioids when indicated because of fear that they may be criticized or, worse, have their licenses revoked for improperly prescribing narcotics. However, *with proper documentation* of relevant history, physical exam, diagnosis, indication for therapy, and response to therapy, there is little to fear. Triplicate prescriptions, where still required, and local institutional policies regarding order and prescription renewal are significant barriers to proper opioid use. However, these should not limit the use of opioids when they are truly indicated.

Finally, some may be reluctant to use opioids, as they may wish to save the "big guns" for later. While tolerance to opioids does exist, it is not a major problem and usually occurrs in patients who require large doses of opioids. For most patients tolerance is not a problem at all. Many patients are successfully maintained on a steady dose of opioids for months to years. When patients complain of increased pain on opioids, it usually reflects worsening underlying disease. Equally important, there is no absolute dose ceiling for opioids (unlike acetaminophen, aspirin, and NSAIDs). Some patients may require and do quite well on the equivalent of more than 100 mgs of IV morphine an hour.

Palliative Care Note

Increased pain in a patient on opioids usually indicates worsening underlying disease, not tolerance.

Specific Opioids

Available medications can be classified by their durations of action. Short-acting opioids can be administered alone or in combination with another analgesic, most commonly acetaminophen. Long-acting medications either have a long serum half-life or a delivery vehicle that allows less frequent administration. A distinction between "strong" and "weak" opioids is less useful. Opioids are similarly efficacious when given in adequate doses.

Short-acting agents are useful for the treatment of rapidly changing pain, such as acute pain and bursts of pain that occur with chronic pain. A short half-life allows rapid titration both up and down. The disadvantages of these agents also relate to their short half-lives. Frequent administration, if given around the clock, can make compliance difficult. Rapid changes in serum drug levels occur. Certain side effects, such as sedation, nausea, and euphoria, are more strongly related to changes in serum levels than to absolute blood levels. Thus, when taken intermittently patients may experience proportionately more side effects with these agents than with comparably dosed long-acting agents.

Long-acting agents either have long half-lives (methadone) or mechanisms for sustained delivery of a short-acting agent (sustained release morphine, hydrocodone, or oxycodone and fentanyl patches). Sustained-release preparations have the advantage of allowing more frequent titration of doses (as the agents' pharmacologic half-lives are short) with the convenience of infrequent dosing. Sustained-release preparations may be safely adjusted after 24 hours. They also may result in smoother opioid blood levels, thereby minimizing side effects.

Morphine

Morphine can be given as soluble tablets, as an elixir, as rectal suppositories, subcutaneously (SC), intravenously (IV), and intramuscularly (IM). While the elixir form is convenient for patients unable to swallow pills, its bitter taste is a problem for some. Morphine has a strong "first pass effect" when given orally. Thus, the oral to parenteral potency ratio is given as 6:1 for a single dose. With chronic administration, this first pass effect lessens, and the oral to parenteral potency ratio is 3:1. It is metabolized in the liver and excreted with active metabolites by the kidneys. The metabolite morphine 6-glucuronide's half-life is particularly prolonged in renal failure. Thus, kidney failure can result in significant drug accumulation of this active metabolite.[18] Although controlled studies comparing different opioid use in renal failure have not been done, many experts recommend that morphine be avoided in such cases.[19] Morphine can cause histamine release, resulting in itching or, rarely, more severe allergic symptoms, although the extent to which this occurs more frequently than with other opioids is debated.[9,20-22] As Katcher notes, the mechanism of morphine-related itching may not always be due to histamine release.[23]

Although histamine release can be a mechanism of true allergy to morphine, more common and clinically important is a "psychological allergy." Having vomited in the past with morphine or simply out of a fear of the drug's reputation, certain patients are very resistant to the use of morphine. In such cases alternatives should be tried.

Tablet sustained-release (SR) morphine is regular morphine given in a slow-release pill form. Because the morphine is in a special waxlike matrix, these pills cannot be crushed, which limits their use in patients who cannot take pills. The lowest dose available is 15 mg. They can be given two to three times a day. The great advantage of these agents is that they combine the best of both worlds: a pharmacologically short serum half-life and twice daily or TID administration. This allows rapid titration of dose. Slow release morphine is relatively inexpensive compared to short-acting morphine.

Kadian is a new form of SR morphine in capsule form with morphine placed inside very small polymeric beads (20 to 100 mg).[24] It is possible to give Kadian capsules only once a day, although patients may require BID dosing. Kadian is expensive but may offer an advantage when enteral morphine administration is desired and patients are unable to swallow pills. The capsule can be opened and sprinkled onto food, such as applesauce, or the beads may be flushed through a gastric-tube. Because of the expense involved, for stable pain methadone, which can be administered as a liquid, is generally preferred in such situations (see below).

If a patient taking slow release morphine becomes nauseated for whatever reason or is unable to take the medication orally, SR morphine can be administered rectally with approximately 90% to 100% of oral efficacy.[9] This may be of help in an emergency. Because of possible discomfort, long-term SR morphine via the rectum is not usually recommended.

Palliative Care Note

In an emergency with patients on SR morphine who become unable to swallow, the tablet can be administered rectally with reasonable absorption, allowing time for clinicians to identify an alternate delivery route.

Generally speaking morphine is the drug of choice for parenteral administration unless side effects become apparent or very high doses (usually greater than 30 mg/h) are to be given subcutaneously (as the volume of administration may become too great for efficient SC administration).

Hydromorphone

Hydromorphone is similar to morphine in duration of action but is approximately five to seven times as potent. When administered orally it can be given in pill form, as an elixir, or as a rectal suppository. An advantage of hydromorphone is that the name does not evoke the strong emotional reactions of morphine.

Hydromorphone is the drug of choice for subcutaneous administration of a high dose of opioid, as it can be delivered in a very concentrated form. It is also the drug of choice when using parenteral opioids in a patient with renal failure or when rotating a patient who is experiencing agitation and myoclonus off morphine.

A slow-release formulation of hydromorphone is available in some countries (not yet the United States). It may serve as a useful alternative to morphine and oxycodone. Angst demonstrated that this agent is effective, although the time to peak-effect is prolonged, approximately 9–12 hours, significantly longer than sustained release morphine or oxycodone preparations (3–6 hours).[25,26]

Oxycodone

Short-acting forms of oxycodone (without acetaminophen) are now available in pill and liquid form. Oxycodone is approximately 1.5 times as potent on a milligram to milligram basis compared to chronic use morphine. It is more expensive than morphine.

SR oxycodone is quite similar to SR morphine in dosage and dosing intervals. SR oxycodone 10 mg q12h is roughly the same as two Percocet tablets (5mg oxycodone/325mg acetaminophen strength) spread over 12 hours. Histamine release appears to be less of a problem than with morphine. Oxycodone should be considered for patients who experience pruritus on morphine and when an oral SR agent is needed in the presence of significant renal failure. It has been argued that oxycodone produces fewer mental status changes than does morphine. This may be a reason for using the drug when mental status changes are attributed to morphine.[27] Other studies have not demonstrated significant differences in side effects between long-acting oxycodone and morphine.[28] However, large controlled trials of the two situations in which an advantage for oxycodone over morphine has been suggested (in significant renal failure and in patients with delirium or at very high risk for delirium) have not been performed.

Palliative Care Note

When ordering SR morphine or oxycodone, write the dosing interval as "q12h," not "BID." (In many institutions BID medications are not given q12h.

SR oxycodone can offer a great psychological advantage in overcoming "opioid-phobia" in patients and health care providers. It may be easier to achieve compliance if it is explained that it is the same active ingredient found in Percocet. The oxycodone is just "spread out" over 12 hours. Unfortunately, there have been reports in the United States of SR oxycodone becoming a drug of choice for opioid abusers, who crush the drug and then take it. Pharmacologically, I know of no reason why oxycodone would have any more or less addictive potential than does any other opioid. Thus, a new wave of opioid-phobia is arising in response to this recent fad of addicts, which may inappropriately limit the use of this agent when otherwise indicated. SR oxycodone is significantly more expensive than is SR morphine. Its use instead of morphine should be justified on a case-by-case basis.

Methadone

Methadone has a long half-life, which allows it to be used on a BID or TID schedule for most patients. It can be given in liquid form and is thus useful in patients who have an enteral route of administration when they are unable to take pills or have a feeding tube. Methadone is cheap. The major problem with methadone is its long half-life. It cannot be rapidly titrated up or down, as it takes days to achieve stable serum levels. Thus, methadone is not indicated in the treatment of rapidly changing pain. Low-dose methadone can be an excellent and inexpensive agent for patients with stable, low-grade, chronic pain. As a rule of thumb, the dose of methadone should not be increased any more rapidly than every three days to avoid possible stacking of doses.* In addition to direct opioid receptor agonist effects, methadone blocks n-methyl-D-aspartate (NMDA) receptors, which may be helpful in refractory pain syndromes.[29,30]

Considerable controversy has arisen regarding conversion ratios for methadone. Recently experts have noted a useful principle: the *higher* the dosage of the opioid being converted *to* methadone, the *lower* the conversion methadone dose should be.[30,31] As summarized by Ripamonti, "The results of our study confirm that methadone is a potent opioid, more potent than believed. Caution is recommended when switching from any opioid to methadone, especially in patients who are tolerant to high doses of opioids."[31]

Palliative Care Note

Do not increase the dose of methadone any more rapidly than every three days in order to avoid the risk of dose-stacking.

Fentanyl Patches

Fentanyl patches may be useful for patients with chronic, stable pain who cannot use the oral route for opioid administration. Patches should not be used for acute pain or in very unstable situations (rapidly escalating or de-escalating pain). Fentanyl has a very short half-life. Transcutaneous patches allow a noninvasive, nonenteral route of opioid delivery, which can be very useful. Serum blood levels remain stable, allowing consistent analgesia and minimizing side effects. Fentanyl patches are expensive. The lowest-dose patch, 25 micrograms per hour, changed every 72 hours, is too strong for some milder chronic pain syndromes. The patches work poorly on very hairy or oily skin. Some patients become allergic to the patches. Absorption increases with increased skin temperature, as with fever, which can be a problem for patients with temperature spikes.[32] Additionally, there are anecdotal reports of decreased absorption (and analgesia) with hypothermia, as is commonly present in the dying process. The clinical significance of these temperature effects is debatable. Further research is needed. Although the drug has a short half-life, it takes approximately 12 to 16 hours to build a reservoir of the drug in the subcutaneous fat when initiating therapy and somewhat longer for the drug to wear off when discontinuing the patch. Caution should be exer-

---

*This rule of thumb assumes simple escalation of methadone. Various schemes for converting other opioids to methadone have been described, including gradual daily decreases in prior opioid doses and daily equivalent increases in methadone over a period of days. (As described in a talk by L. Friedman, "Using Methadone," American Academy of Hospice and Palliative Medicine National Conference, June 2001).

cised during initiation and discontinuation of therapy with this drug. On initiation care must be taken to ensure adequate analgesia until the patch "kicks in." If a long acting opioid, such as SR morphine, is given at the time the patch is placed, this is usually adequate, as this dose will last approximately 12 hours. Otherwise, short-acting agents, such as subcutaneous injections, must be given. Patches cannot be cut in half to reduce the dosage.

Tramadol

Recently available tramadol is an opioidlike drug that binds mu receptors, as do opioids. This drug is unique in that it also blocks reuptake of serotonin and norepinephrine in the CNS. Such reuptake inhibition is a coanalgesic effect to opioid receptor blockade. This inhibition is believed to be partially responsible for the analgesic properties of the drug. Initially, it was thought to have less potential for abuse and to cause fewer side effects. However, with more widespread use concerns have arisen as to abuse potential, and other common opioid side effects have been observed. This drug is more expensive than are traditional agents, and thus routine use is not encouraged. It may be considered in cases with special concerns regarding constipation or respiratory depression.[33]

Opioid Combinations

Combination medications, such as acetaminophen with codeine, oxycodone, or hydrocodone, are similar in terms of duration of action. They differ in terms of opioid potency and coanalgesic dose (acetaminophen or aspirin). Oxycodone (in Percocet, Percodan) appears roughly equipotent and similar in action to hydrocodone (in Vicodin), although good bioequivalent studies for hydrocodone have not been done. However, Vicodin contains 500 mg of acetaminophen, compared to 325 mg in Percocet. These medications are effective when a short-acting agent is needed for mild to moderate pain. Their use is limited by the addition of acetaminophen or aspirin, which are toxic in high doses. Acetaminophen and aspirin as antipyretics may also mask fevers in cases when it would be important to identify a fever, such as immunosuppressed states and postoperatively. Various formulations are available in both pill and elixir forms. Generic formulations, when available, are less expensive.

Acetaminophen with codeine is probably the most commonly used combination analgesic. Codeine is both a direct analgesic, weakly binding mu receptors, and a prodrug. It is converted into morphine in the liver. Patients deficient in a converting enzyme, CYP2D6 (10% of population) or those taking inhibitors of this enzyme, (examples are quinidine, cimetidine and fluoxetine), may not achieve analgesia because of an inability to convert codeine to morphine.[34] Such patients may experience relief with other agents, such as acetaminophen with oxycodone.

Perhaps the biggest problem associated with these drugs is that many physicians will not prescribe stronger opioids when needed if the patient is receiving a maximum dosage of a combination drug. Whether this is out of ignorance, fear, or, at times, laziness is hard to say. I think of this barrier to better pain relief as "the combo wall." However, the barrier exists only in the mind of the prescribing physician. It is very easy to get over this wall—just use an opioid without acetaminophen. For example, if using oxycodone with acetaminophen, simply give pure oxycodone in either a long- or short-acting formulation and continue to titrate up the drug as needed. In the United States certain combo drugs such as hydrocodone and acetaminophen have a lower level of regulatory control. In some states, special prescriptions, triplicates, are required when prescribing a pure opioid. Although using triplicates, where necessary, is a nuisance, it seems inexcusable to deny patients pain relief if needed because of the hassle involved in filling out these forms.

Meperidine (Demerol)

Meperidine has few, if any, advantages over morphine. Meperidine is different in subtle ways from other opioids (greater smooth muscle relaxing effects related to anticholinergic effects, less anti-tussive effect), but these offer no definitive advantages. If given, meperidine should be given IM or IV, not SC, as it is irritating.[9] Meperidine has a toxic metabolite, normeperidine, with a longer half-life than meperidine, which can cause altered mental status, myoclonus, and seizures. This is particularly true in the presence of decreased renal function. Meperidine should not be used for more than 72 hours, not for chronic pain, and *never* in the presence of renal failure.

Propoxyphene (Darvon, Darvocet)

I can think of no reason why propoxyphene-containing agents would be drugs of choice. The analgesia provided is not superior to that of other agents, and there may be a greater potential for side effects associated in part with the accumulation of norprorpoxyphene, a metabolite that can cause cardiac toxicity.[35] The half-life of propoxyphene is 12 to 15 hours and is 30 to 36 hours for norpropoxyphene. Because of these prolonged half-lives, it takes two to three days to achieve steady state serum levels.[9] Thus, there is a potential for dose-stacking, as with methadone.

Medications for Neuropathic Pain

As a rule, treatment of neuropathic pain is more difficult than is treatment of nociceptive pain. Referral to a specialist should be considered if the basic measures outlined below are not successful. Physicians should also be reminded that some neuropathic pain (especially when mixed with nociceptive pain) *may* respond to the agents discussed above, NSAIDs and opioids. However, these agents are less effective for pure neuropathic pain than they are for nociceptive pain.

Three major classes of medication are commonly used in the treatment of neuropathic pain: antidepressants, especially tricyclics; anticonvulsants, especially gabapentin and carbamazepine; and sodium channel blockers, especially mexiletine. A primary care provider may initiate tricyclics, carbamazepine, or gabapentin. Most primary care providers should seek consultation before using other anticonvulsants or sodium channel blocking agents. As a special case, neuropathic pain caused by tumor-related nerve compression is often relieved by steroids by alleviating swelling around the tumor, thereby reducing compression and pain. Dexamethasone 4–8 mg qd. is often effective.

Antidepressants

The analgesic properties of these agents appear to relate primarily to their ability to block neuronal reuptake of serotonin and norepinephrine in the CNS. The anticholinergic properties of tricyclics *do not* appear to have analgesic effects. It is therefore curious that the most anticholinergic agent of available tricyclics, amitriptyline, is used most frequently by physicians for neuropathic pain. This is probably because it is the oldest agent. Agents with less anticholinergic effects, such as nortriptyline and desipramine, should be considered. (Note: these agents may still cause hypotension and should not be used in patients with heart block.) Tricyclics have been used particularly for dysesthetic and constant neuropathic pain, such as diabetic neuropathy. However, they can be used successfully for more paroxysmal pain, such as trigeminal neuralgia. There appears to be a dose–response curve in the use of these agents. While therapy should generally be initiated at low doses (10–25 mg for most tricyclics), dosage should be slowly raised to therapeutic levels (usually 75 mg) or until unacceptable side effects appear if pain relief is inadequate.[9]

Newer antidepressants, such as serotonin reuptake inhibitors (fluoxetine, sertraline), have been inconsistent in their analgesic properties and are not recommended for analgesia. The reason for this lack of analgesia is puzzling and not known.

Anticonvulsants

Most anticonvulsants have been found to have some analgesic effect on neuropathic pain.[36] The most studied is carbamazepine. It has been most commonly used in paroxysmal pain syndromes, such as trigeminal neuralgia, although efficacy has also been demonstrated in more constant pain syndromes, such as diabetic neuropathy. In choosing between a tricyclic and carbamazepine as a first-line agent, it would be reasonable to consider the "two-for-the-price-of-one" principle. Depressed patients with either steady or paroxysmal pain may do better with a tricyclic (barring contraindications). A patient with seizures may better benefit from carbamazepine.

Carbamazepine can be sedating. Patients treated with it should have complete blood counts (CBC) and liver function tests monitored, as blood dyscrasias and LFT abnormalities can occur. These generally resolve with discontinuation of the drug. In patients prone to blood dyscrasias or liver abnormalities, carbamazepine should be used with caution, if at all.

A new anticonvulsant, gabapentin, is increasingly used in the treatment of neuropathic pain.[37–39] It is remarkably well tolerated, with some evidence of anxiolytic effects, and therefore may be helpful for anxious patients.[40,41] Unlike carbamazepine, it lacks significant drug–drug interactions. Patients may experience nausea, especially with rapid dose escalation, or dizziness with higher doses. I have noticed a tendency recently for physicians to prescribe gabapentin in very low doses, 100 mg qhs, for example. Gabapentin is an expensive drug. It makes no sense to prescribe this drug in dosages that virtually prohibit any efficacy. When used, the dosage should be titrated up to therapeutic levels and the patient observed for a clinical response. If unresponsive, the medication should be discontinued.

Routes of Opioid Administration

I turn now to a more detailed discussion of the use of opioids. As mentioned in the section on pain strategy, having considered specific side effects to be avoided and "two-fers," the route of therapy is usually a key consideration in choosing a particular agent.

Oral Route

Generally, the oral route is the preferred route of administration. It is easy to use, and medications are generally cheaper. The oral route also maximizes patient autonomy. It works poorly if patients have trouble swallowing, are intermittently nauseated, or need rapid onset of analgesia. Patients on oral opioids who have nausea and vomiting may have a particularly difficult time reaching a steady state of opioid blood level, which perpetuates nausea. Confused patients and patients dependent on others for administration may have difficulty complying with oral regimens, especially if short-acting agents are relied upon.

Short-acting oral agents, which generally take an hour to reach peak effect, do not work as fast as parenteral agents, which may be a disadvantage if rapid analgesia is desired. This delayed time to peak effect risks slow titration to adequate analgesia or (if additional doses are given prior to peak effect) a "stacking" of multiple doses, resulting in overdosage. On the other hand, use of oral agents, especially long-acting opioids, may avoid possible toxicities associated with rapid increases in blood opioid levels. Some patients may prefer equianalgesic parenteral doses of drugs, believing a shot or injection is more potent. As injections usually take more work on the part of the administrator or nurse, a preference for parenteral injections may reflect a desire for more hands on *care*. I have noticed this tendency particularly in fearful and isolated dying patients.

Enteral Tubes

Nasogastric (NG), percutaneous endoscopically placed gastrostomy (PEG) tubes, and jejunal (J) tubes, if already present, may also be used for drug delivery. These tubes overcome the inability of patients to swallow. More noxious agents, such as concentrated liquid morphine, which is bitter, can be easily administered. Absorption of some drugs may be limited if the patient is vomiting or has significant intestinal obstruction. Probably the greatest problem associated with tubes is the administration of long-acting opioids. SR opioids, such as SR morphine and SR oxycodone, cannot be crushed, as to do so would release the total drug in a short-acting and excessively strong form. Methadone in liquid form or Kadian (morphine in polymeric bead form, which is expensive) can be used if administration of a long-acting agent by tube is desired.

Transdermal Route

Currently, the only major opioid available by the transdermal route is fentanyl. The transdermal route is useful when the enteral route cannot be used. Nauseated patients, patients with poor compliance, and patients unable to swallow are all potential candidates. It takes at least 12 hours (12 to 22 h) for fentanyl to work by the transdermal route. When removed, serum levels fall, on average, 50% in 17 hours.[42] Because of this slow onset and offset of serum levels, fentanyl is useful only for stable, chronic pain and should not be used to treat acute pain. Transdermal fentanyl also works poorly for patients who have very high opioid needs (generally above 500 mcg/h—five 100 mcg/h patches), as patients tend to have difficulty tolerating more than five patches. Transdermal fentanyl is relatively expensive compared to long-acting oral opioid preparations.

Transmucosal

Fentanyl is now available as a lozenge that can be administered through the buccal mucosa. Although expensive, this approach allows rapid onset of analgesia (about 20 minutes) without parenteral administration.[43]

Aerosol

Used primarily in the treatment of dyspnea, opioids administered by a nebulizer can allow rapid peak blood levels, comparable to parenteral administration.[44] Bioavailability via this route is a subject of debate. It would be safest to assume a high degree of bioavailability and then titrate the medication up, based on patient response. Only IV preparations are used for aerosols, with similar peak levels to those obtained using IV administration. Morphine is most commonly used. Care must be taken as, morphine can theoretically release histamine locally, causing bronchospasm, although the clinical significance of this is debatable. I have not seen a patient in which this has happened. All patients I have treated via this route tolerated morphine via other routes without pruritus. It may be wise to give patients who have not previously taken morphine a test dose via another route before giving aerosolized morphine.

Parenteral Administration of Opioids

Parenteral administration of opioids should be considered when:

1. Other routes of administration, especially oral, are not feasible.
2. Rapid dose titration is desired.
3. Very high doses are required.
4. Pain is very unstable, requiring rapid adjustments up and down.

Intravenous Route

The IV route allows the most rapid administration of opioids. This may be useful if rapidly titrating doses is necessary or in treating acute pain. IV administration of opioids offers little, if any, advantage over the SC route. In a prospective cross-over study patients were given IV and SC morphine infusions. There was no significant difference in perceived analgesia between the two routes or in side effects.[45] For practical purposes IV and SC doses are equivalent. The IV route does have a slightly faster onset of action by a few minutes. For very rapid dose titration this may be an advantage. The IV route may be used if an IV is otherwise necessary or if long-term IV access is available—via a

MediPort or percutaneous intravenous catheter (PIC) line, for example. Rarely should an IV be placed simply for the management of chronic pain. The SC route is safer and better tolerated and provides equivalent analgesia.

Intramuscular Route

Opioids may be given via the IM route, although in the majority of cases the SC route is less painful and allows adequate absorption. Of commonly used agents, only meperidine (Demerol) must be given IM, as SC administration is irritating.[9] Patients who require large doses of morphine—may also prefer the IM to the SC route, because injection of large volumes may be irritating.

Subcutaneous Route

Opioid administration via the SC route is generally preferred to the IM. It is useful when short-acting agents need to be administered infrequently. For example, many patients who die over 24 to 48 hours and cannot tolerate oral opioids may be adequately managed with SC morphine injections alone or in combination with a nonoral basal medication, such as a fentanyl patch. The SC route is also frequently used for long-term parenteral administration of opioids.

I am amazed and appalled by the resistance of the medical community to the use of this route for both injections and infusions of opioids. SC injections of opioids (into fat) hurt much less than those into deeper, more tender muscle. Consider the irony. The whole idea is to *relieve pain*. Why would clinicians unnecessarily use a more painful route of administration? Demonstrating the power of culture, the environment, and resistance to change, I have noticed some residents I have trained continue to order IM injections when they leave our palliative care ward. When asked about this practice, some have guiltily admitted that they are tired of being hassled when ordering opioids via the SC route by other members of the health care team, attending physicians, nurses, and pharmacists, who question this behavior. While I am sympathetic to the pressure they may experience, courage is encouraged. Almost all of us will be in an emergency room somewhere, someday and require an opioid injection. Personally, I would like a doctor with the courage to do what is right for me (and is less painful), despite what others might say. (This anecdote also highlights the importance of improving education across the spectrum of health care disciplines. It is not enough just to train physicians.)

Continuous SC infusion of opioids (possible with all but meperidine) offers the following advantages:

1. Ease and comfort of starting infusion: SC infusion needles are quickly and easily inserted into SC fat, either in the abdomen or thigh. Unlike IVs, it is impossible to miss. Insertion is far less painful.

2. Lower infection rate: Relative to IVs, complications, especially infections, are far less common. SC needles are often changed every three days, but may stay in for up to a week.

3. Greater freedom of movement: SC pumps are often small and may be worn on a belt. As the arms are not used, patients may use their arms more freely, maximizing their independence of movement.

Problems with subcutaneous infusions

The major problem with SC infusions is that irritation of the subcutaneous tissue is often volume related. As a rule of thumb, if more than 3 cc's per hour are infused, irritation and pain may be experienced.

A problem can arise when high doses of opioids are needed and the SC route is desirable. It may be difficult to administer morphine, for example, if more than 30 to 40 mg per hour are required. Switching to the more potent hydromorphone, which may be delivered in concentrations as high as 10 mg/cc (equivalent of 50 to 70 mg of morphine/cc), will allow most patients to be successfully treated using the subcutaneous route.

Principles of Basal and Breakthrough (Incident) Drug Dosing

Having determined the opioid to be used and the route of administration, the next questions that usually arise are, "What basal (around-the-clock) drug dose should I prescribe, and what breakthrough (short-acting) drug should I prescribe for breakthrough, or incident, pain?" Much of the art of good pain medication prescription lies in calculating the relative basal and breakthrough doses.

Most patients who have chronic pain require around-the-clock drug dosing. How does one determine the relative basal and breakthrough doses? The following principle is helpful: the more chronic the pain, the more one should rely on the basal dose; the more acute (or unstable) the pain, the more one should depend on the breakthrough, or short-acting, dose.[46]

Palliative Care Note

The more *chronic* the pain, the more one should rely on the basal dose. The more *acute*, or unstable, the pain, the more one should rely on the breakthrough, or short-acting, dose.

In treating chronic, relatively stable pain, a good rule of thumb is that the breakthrough dose should be at approximately that dose that will double the serum opioid level over the basal level when the peak effect has been obtained. This is because a 100% increase (doubling the dose) is usually quite safe. The total dosage of breakthrough medication taken in 24 hours should rarely exceed the 24 hour basal dose in chronic, stable pain. If it does exceed this (or whenever very frequent dosing is given), the basal dose usually needs to be increased. Breakthrough doses should be administered at intervals such that the peak effect of the drug given via a certain route occurs before the next possible breakthrough dose. It is unnecessary and undesirable to schedule breakthrough doses based on the duration of action of the drug. For short-acting oral opioids, such as morphine, the peak effect occurs in approximately one hour. The duration of action of oral morphine in most patients is four hours. Generally, oral morphine as a breakthrough drug should be dosed q1–2 hours, not q4 hours. SR oral opioids usually show a peak effect in three to six hours. IV peak effects correlate with lipid solubility. Peak effect is usually seen in 10 to 15 minutes for morphine. For SC/IM administration, peak effect may occur somewhat later than that for IV. Transmucosal fentanyl demonstrates peak plasma levels in approximately 20 minutes.

Palliative Care Note

Breakthrough doses should be ordered at time intervals slightly longer than the time to peak effect.

The importance of this principle can be appreciated by considering "standard medical practice" in many hospitals and nursing homes. Most clinicians still order oral short-acting opioids every four to six hours PRN pain. Consider this practice more closely. Most short-acting oral opioids do last approximately four hours, assuming normal pharmacokinetics. Dosing every six hours makes no sense, as the drug has worn off significantly by that time. *If* the patient required exactly the prescribed opioid dose every four hours to relieve pain and *if* nursing staff administered the opioid exactly at four hours, then adequate analgesia would be achieved. However, q4h dosing effectively prohibits drug titration against pain, given the drug lasts only four hours. Nurses (and other care providers) often cannot respond immediately at four hours to administer a new dose. Delays of 30 to 60 minutes are not uncommon. During this time the drug may wear off. The peak effect of the new dose will not occur for another hour. The chance of inadequately treated pain in this gap increases substantially. Of course, patients should not generally require opioids as frequently as every one to two hours. If this does occur, it means that either the drug dose is too low or adjustments must be made in basal drug dosing. I suspect the bad habit of prescribing short-acting oral opioids q4–6h arose both from a misunderstanding that stressed dosing based on duration of action, not peak effect, and from concerns about acetaminophen or aspirin toxicity if combination drugs were being used. The misunderstanding can be addressed through education.

Palliative Care Note

For stable, chronic pain a breakthrough dose should roughly double the serum opioid level when peak effect is achieved.

In very unstable, or acute, pain situations it is often appropriate to use no basal dose or to rely primarily on short-acting breakthrough doses. As pain stabilizes and comes under control (and if pain persists in a chronic form), the daily dosage of the short-acting agent used can be of help in calculating a new basal drug dose. The key to appropriate management is flexibility and frequent reevaluation.

When raising the basal dose, it is important to remember to increase by percentage, not milligram. At a minimum an increase should be 25% of the prior dosage. Commonly, the dose is increased by 25% to 100%. In higher dose ranges, physicians tend to underdose because they often increase dosages by milligrams. For example, many physicians are quite comfortable increasing morphine from 2 to 4 mg per hour (a 100% increase of 2 mgs) but will seriously underdose in increasing a patient from 20 mg to 22 mgs (a 10% increase of 2 mgs).

Palliative Care Note

Increase drug doses (by any route) by percentage, not milligram.

Many times I have made the mistake of dutifully increasing the basal drug dose while ignoring the breakthrough dose. For example, 10 mg of morphine may have been a reasonable breakthrough dose when the patient was on 30 mg of sustained-action morphine q12h, but it is clearly inadequate if the basal dose has risen to 90 mg q12h. It is important to remember to adjust breakthrough doses in parallel to basal doses.

Parenteral Basal/Patient Controlled Analgesia Dosing

Most infusion systems allow settings for both basal and patient controlled analgesia (PCA) opioid doses.° Basal doses are set as X mg/h. PCA doses are ordered as Y mg qZ minutes. For SC systems, breakthrough intervals should be no more often than q15 minutes. Every 20 to 30 minutes may be preferable to ensure adequate drug delivery before giving an additional dose.

°Patient controlled analgesia (PCA) refers to a particular type of breakthrough dosing used when a predetermined parenteral drug dose is injected following the push of a button. In reality not all "PCA" breakthrough doses are controlled or administered by patients, who may be physically or mentally impaired. Clinicians or families may administer the breakthrough dose in such cases, which is still often (erroneously) called the "PCA" dose. Thus, in practice parenteral breakthrough doses, when programmed by a pump are often referred to as PCA doses, regardless of who administers the dose.

Once a steady-state basal dosage has been determined, the PCA dosage and interval can be calculated. For stable, chronic pain in accord with the palliative care note above, a good dose is often one that results in a doubling of the serum opioid blood level with peak effect. Dosing intervals should be set such that stacking of PCA doses does not occur. Thus, a patient on 6 mg basal SC morphine might have 2 mg q20 minutes ordered for a PCA dose. In contrast, if a patient is unable to push the PCA button (due to illness or altered mental status, such as dementia), either the basal rate must be emphasized or nursing staff (or family) instructed to assess and administer the PCA dose as needed.

As is true for oral breakthrough doses, patients usually need occasional PCA boluses, but generally these should be less than three to five per day. Such incidents may be anticipated (for example, before nursing care or dressing changes) or unanticipated. If more boluses than this are required, pain should be reassessed and consideration given to raising the basal dose.

It is usually safe to increase the basal dose administered over 24 hours by the amount of PCA doses given over the prior 24 hours. For example, a patient on 6 mg/h basal morphine infusion and a PCA of 2 mg q20 minutes has required 24 injections for a total of 48 mgs of PCA dosing. Dividing this total by 24, this is the equivalent of 2 mg per hour. Thus, at a minimum, the basal dose should be increased by 2 mg/h, from 6 to 8 mg per hour (if pain was well controlled with these PCA doses). If pain was not well controlled with this combination of basal and PCA dosing, a higher basal dose, 10–12 mgs, for example, may be needed.

If *no* PCA boluses are required and the patient is pain free, the basal dose may be too high. This should especially be considered in a patient who appears sedated or talks with slurred speech. If opioid excess is suspected, holding administration of the opioid for a couple of hours and then lowering the dose will usually suffice. Rarely is naloxone administration required. Naloxone should generally be reserved for patients who are beginning to show signs of respiratory depression or hemodynamic compromise, usually associated with bradycardia. Even here, in all but the most extreme cases, consideration should be given to administering small boluses, 0.1–0.2 mg (1/4–1/2 an ampule) incrementally as needed to avoid complete opioid reversal and concomitant pain exacerbation and chemical withdrawal.

Parenteral Basal: PCA Dosing in Unstable and Acute Pain

Unstable pain changes rapidly up and down. Opioids require frequent adjustment. Rapidly lessening pain may be seen in most acute pain syndromes, in which pain naturally decreases over time. Pain following surgery or trauma is usually of this nature. Chronic pain, such as is found in many cancers, may also rapidly decrease in certain situations, such as when a painful focal metastasis is radiated.

When pain is either rapidly increasing or decreasing, proper opioid therapy requires less reliance on basal opioid doses and more on PCA doses. In the extreme, many surgeons treat postoperative pain exclusively with PCA doses. Such therapy has the advantage of minimizing the chance of opioid excess that would result from unnecessary amounts being administered to a patient with lessening pain and a decreasing need for opioids. Excessive reliance on PCA dosing risks making the patient overly dependent on pushing the PCA button on time. Such patients may state that pain is well controlled while awake, but when they fall asleep (and thus cannot push the button) they may suddenly awaken in pain and play "catch-up" with PCA doses. Sleep is thus disturbed, which is an impediment to healing.

Often, what works best in such situations is the use of a PCA:basal hourly ratio that is greater than the 1:1 ratio described for chronic, stable pain. Such a ratio will allow both rapid titration up (in the case of increasing pain) or down.

All machines with PCA:basal drug administration capabilities I have used have a means of recording how many PCA doses were given, when they were given, and often how many attempts were made to administer a dose (a crude measure of desperation). Machines may have a button labeled "history" that allows the clinician to scroll through the PCA history over the past several hours. This data should be used in making adjustments as discussed above.

Conversion among Different Opioids

One would think that converting from one opioid to another would be a simple thing. In theory it is. Just find the right ratio, do the math, and voilà! However, experts disagree on what the appropriate ratios are.[30,47] Recent studies have challenged traditional conversion ratios, which historically were often based on single dose comparisons rather than chronic dosing. Proper conversion is dependent upon a variety of factors—drug dosage, cross-tolerance (or lack thereof) among opioids, and physiologic differences in drug metabolism. As if this were not enough, the *skill* of converting opioids requires more than the use of simple conversion rates. The conversion process must take into account such factors as the amount of residual drug in the patient's system and the time to achieve steady-state blood levels with the new drug as well as individual patient responses during the conversion process. Pereira and Anderson's articles, referenced above, offer excellent recent reviews of controversies in this area for those who wish to pursue further reading. Here, I offer some principles that should help guide conversion efforts:

- When converting from one chronically (around-the-clock) administered opioid to another, first calculate the 24-hour equivalent of the drug from which you are converting. Then convert to the 24-hour equivalent of the new drug (or same drug via a different route of administration) using published conversion ratios.[48]

- Calculate the dosing interval for the new drug.
- Divide the 24 hour dose as appropriate for the new dosing interval. (For example, for q1 hour dosing, divide by 24; for q12 hour dosing, divide by 2.)
- Round off this value (up or down, based on factors such as the quality of pain control at that time and breakthrough drug use.) This dose and dosing interval can serve as the *target* for the new drug, but not usually as the *initial* order in the conversion process.
- Account for residual drug in the patient's system (if any) during the conversion process! This is particularly important if converting from long-acting oral opioids or fentanyl patches. Overdosage may occur if an equivalent dose, based on a conversion table, is used while the old opioid is still in the patient's system. Initiation of the new drug, especially the basal dose, may be delayed if significant residual drug is in the body.

Example. Mr. Smith had been taking sustained-release oral morphine 60 mg q12. His family just managed to get him to take his last oral dose two hours ago. He is admitted to the hospital and can no longer take pills. His pain is well controlled. You wish to start him on a SC (or IV) infusion of morphine. How do you convert to parenteral morphine?

1. Old 24 hour oral morphine dose = 120 mg.
2. Conversion tables show that the oral to parenteral ratio for morphine is 3:1. Therefore, divide 120 mg by 3 to obtain the 24-hour equivalent of parenteral morphine = 40 mg parenteral morphine per 24h.
3. Basal infusions of morphine are written q1h. Therefore divide 40 mg by 24 = 1.66 mg/h.
4. As his pain is well controlled, round-down 1.66 to 1.5 mg/h IV or SC. This is the target basal dose.
5. As approximately 10 hours of sustained-release morphine is in the patient's system, this basal dose should be started in approximately 10 hours. Until then breakthrough doses (approximately 1 mg q30 minutes) may be used. This is the initial drug order.
6. If the patient begins to need frequent breakthrough doses before 10 hours pass, a low basal dose, 0.5–1.0 mg/h, may be initiated based on the reported pain score and breakthrough drug usage. This is the process of adjusting the initial order in the direction of the target order.

- The initial order for the new opioid should have a relatively low basal dose and relatively high breakthrough dose. In calculating a new basal dose, where controversy exists as to the correct conversion value, it is safest initially to use

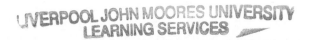

a conversion value that will result in a more conservative (low) new drug dose relative to the old dose. Based on the estimated wash-out period for residual opioids and the individual patient's response in the conversion process, gradually increase the new basal dose, if necessary, based on reported pain scores and the use of breakthrough doses. For example, in converting *from* oral morphine *to* oral hydromorphone, it would be better to use the more conservative ratio (from Table 4.1) of 180 mg morphine: 45 mg hydromorphone. However, if converting *from* hydromorphone *to* morphine, it is safer to use 180 mg morphine: 60 mg hydromorphone, as this will result in a lower initial basal morphine dose.

Palliative Care Note

In the conversion process, depend more on short-acting, breakthrough doses and less on the basal dose. Initially, use a low basal dose of the new drug, adjusting this dose upwards slowly.

The reviews cited above demonstrate that particular caution should be used in converting from one opioid to another at high doses.[30,47] As opioids may differ significantly in terms of their mechanisms of action (for example, methadone's NMDA antagonism) and the degree of cross-tolerance and metabolism, conversion tables may be inaccurate for calculating true equivalent doses, which risks overdosage with the new drug (or occasionally underdosage). This has been found to be particularly true in converting from high doses of opioids such as morphine and hydromorphone to methadone; appropriate morphine-to-methadone ratios tend to be much higher than commonly published ratios.[31,49] That is, a *lower* methadone dose than is suggested by most published tables is appropriate.

TABLE 4.1. 24-Hour Drug Equivalencies of Selected Opioids

DRUG, DELIVERY ROUTE	DOSAGE BY ROUTE
Morphine sulfate, parenteral	60 mg IM, SC, IV
Morphine sulfate, oral	180 mg PO (chronic use)
Methadone	10–40 mg PO
Hydromorphone, parenteral	9–12 mg IM, SC, IV
Hydromorphone, oral	45–60 mg PO
Oxycodone	120 mg PO
Fentanyl	50–100 mcg/h patch (change q72h)
Codeine	1200 mg PO
Hydrocodone	No consensus on equivalent dose

All equivalencies are approximations, *not* starting doses. There is no universal agreement on equivalent doses. Individual dose adjustment is essential!

Recent articles have demonstrated the complexities of opioid conversion and argue against simplistic reliance on tables. Review of these articles is strongly recommended.[30,47] These values are presented as crude guidelines for conversion. As discussed in the text, as important or more important than simply converting milligrams or micrograms is using a protocol that allows adjustment of conversion doses based on individual patient characteristics and responses over time.

Using above values to convert between drugs

1. Calculate current drug 24-h dose (dose times number of times given per day).
2. Multiply this current 24-h dose times the ratio of 24-h equivalent dose of new drug over 24-h equivalent of old drug. This gives 24-h dose of new drug (equivalent doses from table above).

$$\text{current 24-h dose X } \frac{\text{new 24-h equivalent drug dose}}{\text{old 24-h equivalent drug dose}} = \text{new 24-h drug dose}$$

3. Divide new 24-h drug dose by number of times drug to be given per day. This gives new individual drug dose.
4. Order new individual drug dose to be divided per the dosing interval determined above. This is the target dose.
5. Accounting for residual drug in the system, if any, increase new drug toward this target, adjusting as necessary.

Example. Convert sustained-release morphine to parenteral hydromorphone (using conservative conversion—may need to increase hydromorphone later). Current order reads: Sustained-release morphine 60 mg BID.

1. Current 24-h dose is 60 X 2 = 120 mg.
2. 120 mg (old 24-h oral morphine dose) times 9 mg (hydromorphone, parenteral) divided by 180 mg (morphine, oral) = 6 mg/24 h (new dose hydromorphone, parenteral).
3. Divide this 24-h dose by dosing interval—24—for q1 hour basal dose = 0.25 mg/h (hydromorphone, parenteral). This is the target dose.
4. If residual drug is in the patient's system, initially use prn hydromorphone doses. Increase the basal dose based on patient response and prn usage.

Palliative Care Note

When doing conversion calculations, include values such as drug name, administration route, and time intervals in your work. This will protect against serious calculation errors (Fig. 4.4).

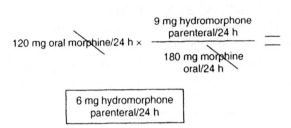

Figure 4.4. Example conversion calculation. Writing in drug name, route, and time intervals in calculations helps avoid serious conversion errors.

Methadone. Considerable controversy has arisen regarding conversion ratios for methadone. Experts have noted a useful principle: The *higher* the dosage of the opioid being converted *to* methadone, the *lower* the conversion methadone dose that should be used. Thus, if a patient were on a high dose of morphine, in converting to methadone I would initially use a conservative 180 mg oral morphine: 10 mg of methadone conversion ratio from Table 4.1. As summarized by Ripamonti, "The results of our study confirm that methadone is a potent opioid, more potent than believed. Caution is recommended when switching from any opioid to methadone, especially in patients who are tolerant to high doses of opioids."[31] I strongly advise using low equivalent doses of methadone initially, gradually increasing the dose while using more liberal doses of breakthrough opioid in the conversion process.

Hydromorphone, parenteral. Controversy exists as to the potency ratio of hydromorphone compared to morphine. Earlier studies suggested that parenteral hydromorphone was seven times as potent as parenteral morphine. More recent studies suggest a 5:1 relative potency.[50] The oral:parenteral ratio for hydromorphone is 5:1 in most tables.

Oxycodone. While American conversion tables have listed oxycodone as being equianalgesic to oral morphine, there is some debate as to equivalency. Some have listed oxycodone as being two times as potent as morphine (Canada). A recent study suggested that oxycodone may be approximately 1.5 times as strong as morphine (Bruera, 1998). Thus, 120 mg of oxycodone is suggested here.

Fentanyl. Fentanyl comes in patches from 25 to 100 ug/h. Patches are changed every 72 hours. A 25 ug/h patch is approximately equal to 50 to 75 mg of oral morphine over 24 h. Levy suggests a simple rule of thumb: that the Fentanyl patch strength (in mcg/h e.g., 25, 50, 100, etc.) is equal to the SR morphine dose given BID.[34] Thus, by this rule a 150 mcg/h patch is equivalent to

150 mg SR morphine q12h. Jannsen, the manufacturer of fentanyl patches, suggests a more conservative dosing schedule in converting to fentanyl patches. Jannsen's dosing table does not allow for a simple conversion value. They suggest a relatively *higher* patch strength at *low* oral morphine equivalents (25 mcg patch for 45–134 mg morphine/24h—consistent with Levy's rule) and a relatively *lower* patch strengths at *higher* morphine doses (200 mcg patch at 675–764 mg morphine/24h—not consistent with Levy's rule). (See manufacturer's product information for details). Their product information stresses that conservative conversion values used for converting *to* fentanyl patches may result in drug overdosage if used to convert *from* patches to other opioids, highlighting the danger of a simplistic use of conversion tables.

Codeine. Although this is the classic conversion value listed in tables, codeine is metabolized into morphine in the liver via the P450 system. About 10% of the population have trouble doing this, and many drugs—for example, Cimetidine and SSRIs—may inhibit this, resulting in even lower potency. Thus actual potency is highly variable.

Hydrocodone. Most conversion tables do not list an equivalent dose for hydrocodone. I have found hydrocodone:oral morphine ratios that range from 6:1 to .75:1 Thus, no recommendation can be given. My impression is that Vicodin (hydrocodone) and Percocet (oxycodone) are very similar in potency.

Special note to teachers of palliative care

Please learn from my mistake! For years I lectured residents and students on principles of pain management along the lines above. Trainees were inspired to go forth and do good deeds. They applauded, I basked in a teacher's glory, and nothing changed. In my teaching I had stressed attitudes (treating pain is important) and knowledge but had underweighted skill training. I found, for example, that most trainees could not use even a basic opioid conversion table (let alone deal with such subtleties as are discussed above). Most residents carried an opioid conversion table in their "peripheral brain"—a small handbook or, recently, a PDA. However, when I asked them to demonstrate the skill of using the conversion table to switch from one opioid to another, they could not. They got confused converting from one drug dosed q12h to another drug dosed TID or q1h. Conversion tables listed an equivalent dose of fentanyl q1 hour, but they could not figure out how this related to the fact that the fentanyl patch is changed q72h. Being unskilled in using tables, they would not use them, fearful of making a mistake (and potentially killing a patient). Thus, it is critical that trainees demonstrate the skills outlined above. Ideally, the practice of such skills will occur in real life under appropriate supervision (as is the case for other medical skills). Barring this, it is strongly recommended that trainees *practice* skills such as opioid conversion using cases in groups or via self-directed learning. Teachers may wish to make up their own cases and ask trainees to perform certain skills (such as writing appropriate opioid orders using a conversion table), or trainees may wish to work independently.

Summary

Pain is a ubiquitous aspect of human experience and epitomizes human suffering. Historically, we have done a poor job of addressing pain. Mercifully, in the majority of cases it can be treated using relatively simple approaches. With a little work we can significantly improve our ability to alleviate the suffering associated with pain.

References

1. Good, M. et al., eds. *Pain as Human Experience*. 1992, University of California Press: Berkeley, p. 1.
2. Portenoy, R. K. and P. Lesage. Management of cancer pain. Lancet 1999; 353(9165): 1695–700.
3. Bonica, J. and J. D. Loeser. Medical evaluation of the patient with pain. In: Bonica J., C. Chapman and W. Fordyce, eds. *The Management of Pain*. 1990, Lea & Febiger: Philadelphia, pp. 563–79.
4. SUPPORT. A controlled trial to improve care for seriously ill hospitalized patients. The study to understand prognoses and preferences for outcomes and risks of treatments (SUPPORT). JAMA 1995; 274(20): 1591–8.
5. Won, A. et al. Correlates and management of nonmalignant pain in the nursing home. SAGE Study Group. Systematic assessment of geriatric drug use via epidemiology. J Am Geriatr Soc 1999; 47(8): 936–42.
6. Grossman, S.A. et al. Correlation of patient and caregiver ratings of cancer pain. J Pain Symptom Manage 1991; 6(2): 53–7.
7. McDowell, I. and C. Newell. *Measuring Health:A Guide to Rating Scales and Questionnaires*, 2nd ed. 1996, Oxford University Press: New York, pp. 355–79.
8. Weissman, D. E. and J. D. Haddox. Opioid pseudoaddiction—An iatrogenic syndrome. Pain 1989; 36(3): 363–6.
9. Twycross, R. *Pain Relief in Advanced Cancer*. 1994, Churchill Livingstone: London, pp. 240, 288, 325, 353, 409–16.
10. Jenkins, C. A. and E. Bruera. Nonsteroidal anti-inflammatory drugs as adjuvant analgesics in cancer patients. Palliat Med 1999; 13(3): 183–96.
11. Hudson, N., A. Taha, et al. Famotidine for healing and maintenance in nonsteroidal anti-inflammatory drug-associated gastroduodenal ulceration. Gastroenterology 1997; 112: 1817–22.
12. Hawkey, C. Cox-2 Inhibitors. Lancet 1999; 353: 307–14.
13. Silverstein, F. E. et al. Gastrointestinal toxicity with celecoxib vs nonsteroidal anti-inflammatory drugs for osteoarthritis and rheumatoid arthritis: The CLASS study:

A randomized controlled trial. Celecoxib Long-term Arthritis Safety Study. JAMA 2000; 284(10): 1247–55.

14. Porter, J. and H. Jick. Addiction rare in patients treated with narcotics [letter]. N Engl J Med 1980; 302(2): 123.

15. Joranson, D. E. et al. Trends in medical use and abuse of opioid analgesics. JAMA 2000; 283(13): 1710–4.

16. Allan, L. et al. Randomized crossover trial of transdermal fentanyl and sustained release oral morphine for treating chronic non-cancer pain. BMJ 2001; 322(7295): 1154–8.

17. Radbruch, L. et al. Constipation and the use of laxatives: A comparison between transdermal fentanyl and oral morphine. Palliat Med 2000; 14(2): 111–9.

18. Mercandante, S. The role of morphine glucuronides in cancer pain. Palliat Med 1999; 12: 182–9.

19. Abrahm, J. A Physician's Guide to Pain and Symptom Management in Cancer Patients. 2000, Johns Hopkins University Press: Baltimore, pp. 135–6.

20. Grossman, S. A. et al. Morphine-induced venodilation in humans. Clinical Pharmacol Ther 1999; 60: 554–60.

21. Warner, M.A. et al. Narcotic-induced histamine release: A comparison of morphine, oxymorphone, and fentanyl infusions. J Cardiothorac Vasc Anesth 1991; 5(5): 481–4.

22. Doenicke, A. et al. Intravenous morphine and nalbuphine increase histamine and catecholamine release without accompanying hemodynamic changes. Clin Pharmacol Ther 1995; 58: 81–9.

23. Katcher, J. and D. Walsh. Opioid-induced itching: Morphine sulfate and hydromorphone hydrochloride. J Pain Symptom Manage 1999; 17(1): 70–2.

24. Broomhead, A. et al. Comparison of a once-a-day sustained-release morphine formulation with standard oral morphine treatment for cancer pain. J Pain Symptom Manage 1997; 14(2): 63–73.

25. Angst, M.S. et al. Pharmacodynamics of orally administered sustained-release hydromorphone in humans. Anesthesiology 2001; 94(1): 63–73.

26. Hanks, G. and N.I. Cherny. Opioid analgesic therapy. In: D. Doyle, G. Hanks, et al., eds. The Oxford Textbook of Palliative Medicine. 1998, Oxford University Press: New York, pp. 331–5, 338–9.

27. Maddocks, I. et al. Attenuation of morphine-induced delirium in palliative care by substitution with infusion of oxycodone. J Pain Symptom Manage 1996; 12: 182–9.

28. Bruera, E. et al. Randomized, double-blind, cross-over trial comparing safety and efficacy of oral controlled-release oxycodone with controlled-release morphine in patients with cancer pain. J Clin Oncology 1998; 6: 3222–9.

29. Mercadante, S. et al. Switching from morphine to methadone to improve analgesia and tolerability in cancer patients: A prospective study. J Clin Oncol 2001; 19(11): 2898–904.

30. Pereira, J. et al. Equianalgesic dose ratios for opioids. A critical review and proposals for long-term dosing. J Pain Symptom Manage 2001; 22(2): 672–87.

31. Ripamonti, C. et al. Switching from morphine to oral methadone in treating cancer pain: What is the equianalgesic dose ratio? J Clin Oncol 1998; 16(10): 3216–21.

32. Southam, M. Transdermal fentanyl therapy: System design, pharmacokinetics and efficacy. Anti-Cancer Drugs 1995; 6(suppl 3): 26–34.

33. Grond, S. et al. High-dose tramadol in comparison to low-dose morphine for cancer pain relief. J Pain Symptom Manage 1999; 18(3): 174–9.

34. Levy, M.H. Pharmacologic treatment of cancer pain. New Engl J Med 1996; 335(15): 1124–32.
35. Ulens, C., P. Daenens, et al. Norpropoxyphene-induced cardiotoxicity is associated with changes in ion-selectivity and gating of HERG currents. Cardiovasc Res 1999; 44(3): 568–78.
36. Tremont-Lukats, I.W., C. Megeff, et al. Anticonvulsants for neuropathic pain syndromes: Mechanisms of action and place in therapy. Drugs 2000; 60(5): 1029–52.
37. Hemstreet, B. and M. Lapointe. Evidence for the use of gabapentin in the treatment of diabetic peripheral neuropathy. Clin Ther 2001; 23(4): 520–31.
38. Garafalo, E. Gabapentin for the symptomatic treatment of painful neuropathy in patients with diabetes mellitus: A randomized controlled trial. JAMA 1998; 280: 1831–6.
39. Kishore, A. and L. King. Fast Fact and Concept #49; Gabapentin for neuropathic pain. End of Life Care Education Project. http://www.eperc.mcw.edu/, 2001.
40. Miller, L.J. Gabapentin for treatment of behavioral and psychological symptoms of dementia. Ann Pharmacother 2001; 35(4): 427–31.
41. Pande, A.C. et al. Placebo-controlled study of gabapentin treatment of panic disorder. J Clin Psychopharmacol 2000; 20(4): 467–71.
42. Hanks, G. and N.I. Cherny. Opioid analgesic therapy. In: D. Doyle, G. Hanks, et al., eds. *The Oxford Textbook of Palliative Medicine*. 1998, Oxford University Press: New York, p. 340.
43. Farrar, J. et al. Oral transmucosal fentanyl citrate: Randomized, double-blinded, placebo controlled trial for treatment of breakthrough pan in cancer patients. J Natl Cancer Inst 1998; 90: 611–6.
44. Chandler, S. Nebulized opioids to treat dyspnea. American Journal of Hospice & Palliative Care 1999; 1999(16): 418–22.
45. Nelson, K. et al. A prospective, within-patient, crossover study of continous intravenous and subcutaneous morphine for chornic cancer pain. J Pain Symptom Manage 1997; 13: 262–7.
46. Portenoy, R.K., ed. Cancer pain management: Update on breakthrough pain. Seminars in Oncology 1997; 24(suppl): 116.
47. Anderson, R. et al. Accuracy in equianalgesic dosing: Conversion dilemmas. J Pain Symptom Manage 2001; 21(5): 397–406.
48. Gordon, D.B. Opioid equianalgesic calculations. Journal of Palliative Medicine 1999; 2(2): 209–18.
49. Ripamonti, C. et al. Equianalgesic dose/ratio between methadone and other opioid agonists in cancer pain: Comparison of two clinical experiences. Ann Oncol 1998; 9(1): 79–83.
50. Lawlor, P., K. Turner, et al. (1997). "Dose ratio between morphine and hydromorphone in patient with cancer pain: a retrospective study." Pain 72(1–2): 79–85.

5

Non-Pain Symptom Management

The stories that ill people tell come out of their bodies. The body
sets in motion the need for new stories when its disease disrupts
the old stories.

> Arthur Frank. *The Wounded Storyteller:*
> *Body, Illness and Ethics*

I was at the movie theater on a Saturday when I received a page about Mr. A.
He was scheduled to be admitted to our hospice ward that coming Monday. I
had not met Mr. A. The resident was very sorry to disturb me, but she needed
to ask, "Can your hospice do IVs and antibiotics?" I sighed quietly, having had
similar discussions many times before. "Yes," I replied, "We can. The question is—would those therapies be helpful relative to what we are trying to do."
The resident explained that Mr. A. had bowel obstruction and was receiving
the usual care. He had a nasogastric tube (NG) in place and an IV running.
His nausea was being treated with lorazepam. The problem was that Mr. A.
wanted to see his son, who was in the Philippines, before he died. There were
visa issues, and it might take a few weeks to get things straightened out. Thus,
the family was interested in keeping him alive until then. Again, the resident
apologized. Life prolongation seemed to be against hospice philosophy, but
the resident asked if we could make an exception in this case given the impor-

tance of the son's visit. Unfortunately, Mr. A. was obtunded, but it would be so important to the family.

I explained that hospice is not opposed to people living longer. *Life* is an important aspect of quality of life, so if there were simple things we could do to increase the chance that Mr. A. would get see his son, this was completely in keeping with hospice philosophy and fine with me. In the meantime, I wondered out loud, would the team be interested in some suggestions for his care. "Please," replied the resident. I suggested that octreotide be added to his drug regimen and that a different antiemetic be used, as lorazepam was likely doing little other than sedating the patient. It was fine to keep the NG and IV in place for now. We would reevaluate their use when he came to hospice.

When he arrived we found Mr. A. sitting up in bed, smiling. "He woke up!" said his wife. His chart revealed that the amount of fluid draining from the NG had decreased dramatically following administration of octreotide. Over the next few days with various interventions we managed to discontinue the NG and the IV. He began to eat despite his continuing obstruction and became ambulatory. He was discharged to home hospice, where he lived for two months until shortly before his death, when he returned to our unit. Unfortunately, his son did not make it in time. However, his family remarked on how precious the extra time at home had been.

I share this story because it illustrates several points. First, palliative care should not be so much about *what* we do (IVs or antibiotics) as about *why* we do it. What is our *intent*, and how does this intent relate to the goals of care established by the patient, family, and clinicians? Second, many view the choice between palliative or hospice care and traditional medical care as being a choice between being comfortable (but inevitably dying sooner) in hospice and living longer, albeit with less comfort, in traditional care. In most cases this is a false choice. There is no good evidence that people, appropriately selected, who elect a palliative approach to care die sooner than do those in traditional care. It is also a false choice in that it implies to some that living longer in hospice is necessarily a bad thing, or at least is antithetical to hospice philosophy, which it is not.

As I will discuss further in the section on bowel obstruction, I believe Mr. A. lived better and longer because he received palliative care. "Standard therapy" for bowel obstruction, including long-term NG suction and IV fluids, may result in patients dying sooner than they would with state-of-the art palliative care. The treatment of Mr. A's nausea with lorazepam was inept and even harmful, but not unusual. Although people are just beginning to understand how little clinicians learn and know about pain management, few are aware that, if possible, ignorance of effective therapies for many non-pain symptoms is even greater than is that for pain.

One day several years ago an intern with whom I was working asked a very simple question. "What is the difference between Phenergan [promethazine] and Compazine [prochlorperazine]?" Although I had been doing palliative care for more than a year, I was embarrassed to admit to her and to myself that I did not know. Hence, I tried to find out. I was shocked to find that these medicines, which I had been using for years almost interchangeably, were almost exact opposites in their pharmacology. I just did not know.

Since then, I am still amazed at how little attention non-pain symptoms receive in medical education. I recall a conference I attended a few years ago. Half the conference was devoted to pain and the other half to various aspects of end-of-life care. I was asked to speak about non-pain symptoms. I thought, "This a peculiar balance—half the conference on one symptom, pain, and a one-hour session on non-pain symptoms." Of course, it was impossible to cover every non-pain symptom in one hour, and it is equally impossible to do justice here to the wide array of non-pain symptoms that may arise. Still, I will highlight some distressing symptoms often encountered in practice.

Nausea and Vomiting

We have all suffered from nausea and vomiting. In the midst of severe nausea, our world view changes to the extent that nausea becomes our dominant experience. Perhaps that is why in English the expression *to be sick* is synonymous with nausea and vomiting. Nausea and vomiting often arise secondarily to other common diseases and as side effects of medical therapy. Despite the totality of suffering engendered by the experience of nausea and vomiting, relatively little attention has been paid to diagnosis and treatment. Most clinicians prescribe medications such as prochlorperazine (Compazine) or promethazine (Phenergan) for nausea of any etiology with a "one size fits all" mentality. In fact, as more is learned about the pathophysiology of nausea and vomiting, the better therapy can be tailored to a specific cause. So doing will allow better palliation and avoid unwanted side effects.

Why Do We Experience Nausea and Vomiting?

Nausea and vomiting, unpleasant as they are, serve important purposes. They protect us from ingesting toxic substances, an evolutionary advantage.* Our senses of sight, smell, and taste can serve to protect us from eating substances

---

*Most animal research on nausea is performed on ferrets, apparently one step up the evolutionary tree from rodents, which do not vomit.

that might be bad for us. A useful rule of thumb is that if something looks gross or smells or tastes awful, it probably is. Unfortunately, looks, smell, and taste can sometimes be deceiving, so we may still eat something poisonous. If ingested, a toxic substance may irritate the stomach or intestine, stimulate special chemoreceptors, and cause vomiting, thus limiting absorption of the poison, but even this is not adequate protection. Some toxins may get through these safeguards. The brain has a variety of receptors that test for potential toxins. Stimulation of these receptors triggers nausea and vomiting, preferably in time to limit further ingestion of poison. Memory also serves as a protective mechanism. If eating something made you sick before, it probably will do so again. The memory of nausea and vomiting associated with that substance would itself be a potent stimulus for nausea, overcoming hunger. In this sense nausea and vomiting helped our species survive over millennia.

Unfortunately, nausea arises with certain illnesses and secondarily to certain therapies in ways that offer no survival advantage. Indeed, nausea and vomiting in such cases may increase the morbidity and mortality of illness through dehydration, electrolyte imbalance, and limitation of food intake.

Pathophysiology of Nausea and Vomiting

Good evidence exists that various stimuli that affect nausea and vomiting come together in an area in the brain known as the vomit (or emetic) center in the medulla. This "center" is not a discrete nucleus, but a complex array of neurons coordinated by a "central pattern generator."[1] Still, for our purpose, it is useful to think of a final pathway that gives rise to vomiting. The vomit center receives input from four major areas: the GI tract, the chemoreceptor trigger zone, the vestibular apparatus, and the cerebral cortex. (The center also has intrinsic chemoreceptors that can modulate, stimulate, and repress nausea.)[2,3] Each of these four areas responds to certain types of stimuli, modulated by specific neurotransmitters that bind specific receptors. Understanding how these areas modulate nausea and vomiting helps us tailor specific therapies for specific problems.

The GI tract

As the primary source of toxin absorption is the gut, the effect of the GI tract on the vomit center is complex. Stimulation of the gut chemoreceptors and stretch receptors triggers nausea and vomiting via vagal nerve afferents and afferent fibers associated with the sympathetic nervous system. Serotonin, acetylcholine, histamine, and substance P are major neurotransmitters involved in stimulating these receptors. Chemoreceptors in the gut appear to be major mediators of the toxic effect of certain chemotherapeutic agents, such as cisplatin, even when such drugs are given intravenously via binding to $5HT_3$ receptors.

In addition to being a neurotransmitter that stimulates nausea, acetylcholine also increases gut motility and gut secretion. Histamine mediates transmission of nausea via the vagus nerve. Substance P binds neurokinin 1 receptors in the gut (and directly in the vomit center in the brain).[4,5]

The chemoreceptor trigger zone (CTZ)

The CTZ senses chemicals in the blood. The CTZ is particularly sensitive to increasing blood levels of potentially toxic substances. If a toxic substance is detected, nausea is experienced and the vomit reflex initiated—hopefully before more toxin is absorbed. It is easy to understand the evolutionary advantage of such a failsafe. The brain detects an "alien" chemical. By itself, this is not so unusual—we have lots of peculiar non-self chemicals floating around in our bloodstreams. However, if the concentration of a chemical is rapidly rising, this could constitute a threat to our health—better to expel any residual substance in the stomach; better safe than dead. Two major neurotransmitters are involved—dopamine, acting on D_2 receptors, and serotonin, acting on $5HT_3$ receptors. Different toxin responses are mediated through different neurotransmitters. Opioid-related nausea appears to be most related to stimulation of D_2 receptors. Understanding this has helped with selective blockage of specific receptors in specific disorders.

The vestibular apparatus

Motion and body position are sensed through the vestibular apparatus. Motion sickness, such as car sickness and seasickness, are mediated through the vestibular apparatus, as are inner-ear diseases, such as Meniere's disease. The vestibular apparatus may once have served as a sensor for certain neurotoxins (such as alcohol) that can produce disequilibrium. Stimulation of the vestibular apparatus by alcohol may provide a survival advantage in keeping our species from, literally, drinking ourselves to death. Stimulus of the vestibular apparatus is mediated largely through histamine and acetylcholine receptors.

The cerebral cortex

The cerebral cortex and associated structures in the limbic system modulate complex experiences such as taste, sight, and smell as well as memory (involved in anticipatory nausea) and emotion. Discrete neuropathways are less well understood. However, higher cortical effects are still important and can be extremely powerful in stimulating and suppressing nausea and vomiting.

Principles of Therapy

It almost goes without saying that if we can find curable causes for nausea (or other symptoms) and can eliminate these causes, this is ideal. However, for many chronic illnesses this is impossible. We often need to treat nausea and vomiting as unavoidable side effects of necessary therapies. Even patients who have acute, self-limited illnesses, like gastroenteritis, want to have their nausea palliated. Fortunately, there is a lot we can do. Therapy will work best if it is tailored to the specific cause (curable or otherwise) of nausea and vomiting.

A useful mnemonic for remembering causes of nausea and vomiting is vomit. Recalling these causes will help to figure out which approaches are best in treating particular patients.

Vestibular
Obstruction (opiates)
Mind (dysmotility)
Infection (irritation of gut)
Toxins (taste and other senses)

Vestibular

Patients who have vestibular involvement may complain of poor balance, nausea stimulated by rapid head movement or motion, and other inner-ear symptoms, such as changes in hearing or ear ringing. Minimizing movement can help to minimize nausea mediated through this system. Medications with strong antihistaminic and anticholinergic properties are most useful. Many medications are available that block both histamine and acetylcholine receptors. All available medications are sedating. Newer nonsedating antihistamines cannot be used because their lack of sedation relates to poor penetration across the blood–brain barrier. Thus, while they are good for blocking histamine receptors peripherally, they are not useful for blocking central receptors.

Obstruction (dysmotility)

Obstruction and poor gut motility result in the back-up of the contents of the gut. Mechanoreceptors and chemoreceptors are stimulated, and nausea is triggered. The more distal the obstruction in the gut, the more the abdomen will be distended and the longer it will take for gut contents to back up. (See the section on bowel obstruction) Obstruction can be mechanical or "functional."* The most common cause of obstruction is constipation. In at-risk patients, this should be ruled out by history, rectal examination, and X-ray examination, if necessary.

A variety of patients are at risk for functional bowel obstruction caused by dysmotility. Diabetics may have gastric neuropathies. Patients on opioids and anticholinergic drugs commonly experience dysmotility of both the upper and lower gut. Patients who have dysmotility often complain less of frank nausea than

---

*A peculiar idiosyncrasy of medical language is the use of the term *functional*, when it in fact refers to a process that is *dysfunctional*. *Functional bowel obstruction* means that despite an obstructive presentation, there is no physical blockage of the intestine (other than by intraluminal contents). In theory, the bowel could function (thus the term), but, in fact, it is dysfunctional.

of early satiety. Classically, they will have a modest appetite, then be able to eat very little, followed shortly by abrupt regurgitation of undigested food. Unless contraindicated (as in Parkinson's disease or advanced renal failure), metoclopramide is the drug of choice for such dysmotility of the upper GI tract. Removing offending agents (such as anticholinergic drugs) may improve dysmotility. Anticholinergic drugs antagonize the activity of metoclopramide and should therefore be decreased or eliminated, if possible, when starting this drug. Metoclopramide binds $5HT_4$ receptors, which in turn release acetylcholine, stimulating motility. Anticholinergic drugs antagonize this effect.

Palliative Care Note

Avoid using anticholinergic antiemetics with metoclopramide, as these antiemetics antagonize the action of this drug.

A common problem in palliative care is the "squashed stomach syndrome." Patients who have enlarged livers due to cancer or hepatitis may present with early satiety and abrupt vomiting in a syndrome clinically indistinguishable from dysmotility as described above.[6] Although technically a form of mechanical bowel obstruction due to extrinsic compression, therapy is identical to that for dysmotility, stressing promotility agents such as metoclopramide.

Mind

The mind can have a powerful effect on the experience of nausea and vomiting. A peaceful environment with appealing sights, smells, and tastes can promote appetite. A lack thereof can cause or exacerbate nausea, as can anxiety and depression. Anxiolytics such as benzodiazepines can be helpful for anxiety and are specifically indicated in anticipatory nausea associated with chemotherapy.[7] (Please note that there is no evidence to support the use of lorazepam as a sole agent for the treatment of nausea outside of these indications. Lorazepam can induce sedation and theoretically increase the risk of aspiration in a sedated vomiting patient. The case of Mr. A. highlights this point.) Depression, when present, should be addressed. Adjusting food presentation for ill patients can be a challenge. Fatty and spicy foods are best avoided. With serious illness tastes may change. In advanced cancer meat is often said to taste bad. Very sweet substances may be poorly tolerated. Slightly sour, cooler, easy-to-digest foods are often best.

Infection/irritation/inflammation

Nausea and vomiting may be a nonspecific sign of an acute gastrointestinal infection and require little more than sympathy and perhaps treatment with anticholinergic/antihistaminic agents, such as promethazine. Irritation of the stomach and intestinal tract may be ameliorated with coating agents, such as sucralfate or bismuth-containing preparations, such as Pepto-Bismol. Nausea may be an early sign of more serious infection, such as pyelonephritis, pneumonia, or CNS infection. These causes should be considered, as appropriate.

Various therapeutic agents and medications can induce inflammation. Inflammation anywhere in the body may result in the release of substances that stimulate nausea through a direct effect on the brain (principally through vomit center receptors, such as neurokinin-1 receptors). Gut inflammation through the use chemotherapeutic agents and radiation therapy is a potent stimulant of nausea. The exact mechanisms through which nausea is stimulated in this way are still being worked out. Preliminary work suggests that serotonin binding of $5HT_3$ receptors and substance P binding of neurokinin-1 receptors may be particularly important. For example, randomized controlled trials have demonstrated superiority for the use of $5HT_3$ antagonists for radiation enteritis.[8–10]

These studies suggest the possibility that when gut inflammation is thought to be a major contributor to nausea, anticholinergic and antihistaminic agents may be fine for minor or self-limited nausea. However, for more severe forms of nausea, $5HT_3$ antagonists may be preferable. Neurokinin-1 antagonists are being developed and may also be helpful for this form of nausea, although they are not yet clinically available.[11]

Toxins

The major toxins of today are not found in strange plants, as was the case for our distant ancestors, but are the medications we give our patients. Many drugs can cause nausea and vomiting as side effects. Most clinicians are quick to suspect opioids, such as morphine. They may forget such common drugs as digoxin, nonsteroidal anti-inflammatory agents (NSAIDs), and newer antidepressants such as fluoxetine (Prozac) or sertraline (Zoloft). New-onset nausea should always prompt a medication review and consideration of withholding possibly offending agents.

Because opioid-related nausea is so common, it will be discussed separately. Opioids result in nausea through two major mechanisms: inhibition of gut motility and stimulation of the CTZ. Stimulation of the CTZ relates more to increases in blood opioid levels than it does to absolute opioid levels. Thus, initiating opioid therapy or raising the opioid dose is likely to result in nausea. However, if a new steady-state blood level is maintained, nausea usually subsides within two to three days. During this time aggressive treatment of nausea usually allows patients to tolerate opioid therapy. This is particularly important if the oral route is used for administration. Patients may enter a vicious cycle of nausea interrupting oral opioid administration, resulting in fluctuating blood opioid levels and perpetual nausea (in addition to unnecessary pain). In severe cases a nonoral route of administration should be used, at least until nausea is under control, in order to escape this cycle. As stimulation of the CTZ is primarily mediated through D_2 receptors, dopamine blockade is critical to drug therapy. Anticholinergic and antihistaminic agents are less effective for this form of nausea, although they may help with relatively minor stimulation of the vestibular apparatus by opioids. Anticholinergic and antihistaminic agents may increase undesired sedation associated with initiation or upward titration of opioids and may also exacerbate poor gut motility, adding to these serious side affects of opioids. Anticholinergic and antihistaminic agents dry the mouth, a common and troubling side effect in the seriously and terminally ill patient (also worsened in patients taking opioids). Thus, a strong argument can be made for maximizing dopamine blocking effects and minimizing anticholinergic and antihistaminic effects in choosing an antiemetic for opioids. Having said this, it is remarkable that no controlled trials (of which I am aware) have compared prochlorperazine (Compazine—relatively antidopaminergic) to promethazine (Phenergan—a weak antidopaminergic drug and strong antihistamine) in the treatment of opioid-related nausea. Given the prevalence with which both agents are used to treat opioid-related nausea, this is testimony to the fact that what often drives research is not solving common, practical problems, but pharmaceutical dollars and research ambitions.

Specific Medications for Nausea

Few randomized control studies have compared specific medications for specific causes of nausea. In particular, little attention has been paid to potential toxicities of specific agents. However, as discussed above, research has progressed in understanding the relationship between receptors and nausea (summarized in Fig. 5.1). Based on in vitro receptor binding, Peroutka and Snyder developed the following table (Table 5.1): (Lower numbers indicate tighter binding and therefore greater blockade of the receptor. Example: Scopolamine is strongly anticholinergic, as it has a very low number, 0.8 for the cholinergic receptor.) Potency: $K1$ (nanomolar).

Scopolamine

As is readily seen, scopolamine is a pure anticholinergic agent. It can be useful in treating motion-related nausea and when sedation or other anticholinergic

TABLE 5.1. Receptor Binding of Common Antiemetics

DRUG GROUP	DOPAMINE 2	MUSC. CHOLINERGIC	H1 HISTAMINE
Scopolamine	>10,000	.08	>10,000
Promethazine	240	21	2.9
Prochlorperazine	15	2100	100
Chlorpromazine	25	130	28
Metoclopramide	270	>10,000	1,100
Haloperidol	4.2	>10,000	1600

Source: Adapted from Peroutka and Snyder.[12]

effects are desired, such as decreasing gut secretions and alleviating cramping due to bowel obstruction. Marketed for motion sickness, scopolamine is available as a patch. It can be given SC. Effects last approximately six hours.

Promethazine (Phenergan)

Promethazine has strong anticholinergic and antihistaminic effects. Its weak binding of dopamine receptors suggests it would be a poor choice as an antiemetic for opioid-related nausea. Despite this, it is commonly used for opioid-related nausea (perhaps based on misguided extrapolations from its use in combination with meperidine and chlorpromazine as a pediatric sedative in emergency rooms).[13] Therefore, promethazine is not recommended for pure opioid-related nausea. It is available in oral, IM, IV, and rectal suppository forms. Promethazine may be a drug of choice when a drug, especially a suppository, is needed for motion-related nausea and when other anticholinergic and antihistaminic effects are desired, as in viral gastroenteritis.

Prochlorperazine (Compazine)

Prochlorperazine has strong dopamine and histamine receptor binding, with weak cholinergic receptor binding. It is mildly sedating. It is available in oral (tab, liquid), IV, IM, and suppository forms. Prochlorperazine can be considered a good choice when a suppository is needed for opioid-related vomiting and anticholinergic effects are to be avoided.

One of the few randomized controlled studies done for nonchemotherapy-related nausea compared promethazine to prochlorperazine for the treatment of "nonspecific" nausea and vomiting in 84 patients in an emergency room. Although the precise causes of such nausea were not given in the study, presumably the majority were self-limited inflammatory states such as viral gastro-

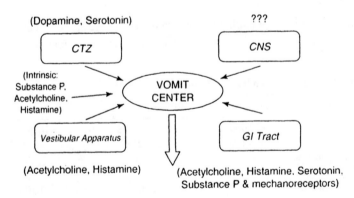

Figure 5.1. A final pathway for nausea.

enteritis. The study found that prochlorperazine was superior to promethazine in a number of regards: (1) superior nausea relief on a visual analogue scale, (2) shorter time to onset, (3) fewer treatment failures, and (4) a superior side effect profile—less sedation and no greater extrapyramidal side effects.[14] These results are striking in that they are contrary to what we might expect based on receptor binding. It is not clear why prochlorperazine, which is principally an antidopaminergic agent, would be superior to anticholinergic, antihistaminic promethazine, because a pharmacologic basis for the efficacy of dopamine blockade in inflammatory forms of nausea has not been described. This highlights the need for clinical studies in this area.

Chlorpromazine (Thorazine)

Like haloperidol, chlorpromazine is most commonly used as an antipsychotic agent. From Table 5.1 it can be seen that this agent has a strong affinity for all three receptors. It is therefore useful in opioid-related nausea as well as in other forms when anticholinergic and antihistaminic effects are desired. However, it should be avoided if sedation is undesirable. It can be given PO, IM, or rectally but should not be given SC. Chlorpromazine also blocks alpha receptors and therefore can cause or exacerbate postural hypotension. Chlorpromazine can, in addition, lower the seizure threshold and thus should be used with caution, if at all, in patients prone to seizures.

Metoclopramide (Reglan)

Metoclopramide has relatively weak binding across the board. Binding is strongest at dopamine receptors, and (not shown here) in high doses it can be effective in blocking $5HT_3$ serotonin receptors. As discussed above, metoclopramide is useful when an upper GI tract prokinetic agent is desired, especially in the presence of opioids. It can be given PO, IV, or via SC infusion.[15]

Haloperidol (Haldol)

Haloperidol has the strongest dopamine receptor binding, with little anticholinergic or antihistaminic effects. It is therefore ideal for opioid-related nausea. It is also useful in the treatment of delirium, dementia, and psychosis when sedation is undesirable. Haloperidol (as with other antidopaminergic agents) is contraindicated in Parkinson's disease. Haloperidol strongly blocks D_2 receptors and has minimal anticholinergic and antihistaminic effects. It is minimally sedating. It can be given PO (tablet or liquid), IM, or by slow SC infusion. Unfortunately, no rectal form is available. Because haloperidol is marketed as an antipsychotic, most physicians are not familiar with the use of haloperidol for nausea despite wide experience in the hospice community with this selective agent.

5HT₃ antagonists

Chemotherapy with certain agents can cause intense nausea largely mediated through $5HT_3$ serotonin receptors, found both in the gut and in the CTZ. These drugs are very expensive and should not be used routinely except for the treatment of chemotherapy-related nausea and in certain special circumstances. This class of drugs may be useful for nausea related to bowel obstruction and may have broader use for inflammatory states involving the bowel, as suggested by data that support their use in radiation enteritis. They have also been found to be helpful in postoperative nausea.[16] They may also be used in CTZ-related nausea when antidopaminergic drugs are strongly contraindicated, as in Parkinson's disease.

Other Agents

Cyclizine and other antihistamines such as meclizine and diphenhydramine are useful in the treatment of motion sickness. Steroids may be considered for nausea related to chemotherapy and radiation therapy.[17] Steroids also actively stimulate the appetite, may be mildly euphoric, and can be helpful in certain pain syndromes. They are helpful, therefore, in a variety of cancer-related conditions but can have serious side effects, especially with prolonged use. The antidepressant mirtazapine may be helpful in treating nausea associated with chemotherapy when $5HT_3$ receptors are being stimulated. It has some blocking activity at such receptors and may also act as an anxiolytic through blockade of $5HT_2$ receptors.[18] Dronabinol and other marijuana related compounds have shown significant efficacy in chemotherapy-related nausea and can increase appetite.[19] Psychological effects associated with this class of drugs may be viewed as beneficial or deleterious (Table 5.2).[19]

Constipation

Constipation is a common problem for many patients.[21-24] Therapy should be individually tailored; what is very good therapy for one type of constipation may be poison for another.[25] It is difficult for young people, who may never have experienced constipation, to relate to the distress caused by this disorder. For those afflicted, the whole tone of the day may be set by the presence or absence of a good bowel movement (BM).

Understanding how a normal BM is created helps us understand how the process can go awry. Our goal in treating constipation is not to "cure" something, it is to help the patient return to the best possible balance that will allow a normal BM to be passed.

TABLE 5.2. Summary table Relating Type of Nausea, Receptor, Drug Class, and Example of Drug of Choice.[20]*

TYPE OF NAUSEA	RECEPTORS CAUSING NAUSEA	DRUG CLASS USEFUL	EXAMPLES OF DOC
Vestibular	Cholinergic, histaminic	Anticholinergic, antihistaminic	Scopolamine patch, promethazine
Obstruction of bowel caused by constipation	Cholinergic, histaminic, ? $5HT_3$	Stimulate myenteric plexus	Senna products
DysMotility of upper gut	Cholinergic, histaminic, ? $5HT_3$	Prokinetics stimulate $5HT_4$ receptors	Metoclopramide
Infection, Inflammation	Cholinergic, histaminic, ? $5HT_3$	Anticholinergic, antihistaminic	Promethazine, prochlorperazine
Toxins stimulating the CTZ in the brain such as opioids	Dopamine 2, $5HT_3$	Antidopaminergic, $5HT_3$ antagonist	Prochlorperazine, haloperidol, ondansetron

*The Fast Fact concept was developed by Dr. Eric Warm. His idea was to distribute brief one- to two-page summaries of important issues in palliative care to physicians-in-training. Under Dr. David Weissman's guidance, more than 60 Fast Facts have been written and are available at: http://www.eperc.mcw.edu/.

Four major components affect the production of a normal BM: solid waste, water, movement, and lubrication. Although we can differentiate these separate components, in fact, they are very much interrelated. For example, decreased movement of intestinal contents allows more water to be absorbed.

Solid Waste

Our bodies cannot absorb everything we eat. We also "create" waste, dead cells and bacteria, within our intestines, which needs to be excreted. Too much or too little solid waste can be a problem. Many people eat little fiber, a major component of solid waste. With little fiber stool volume decreases, and there is less material for the intestinal tract to push along. The intestinal tract becomes sluggish, and with slow passage more water is absorbed. Constipation results, and patients experience small, dry stools. Therapy for such patients is to replace the fiber they do not get in their diets. Psyllium fiber can be useful in this regard. The intestine responds to increased stool volume, within reason, with greater contraction. Thus, bowel contents are moved along more efficiently, and less water is absorbed, resulting in healthy BM.

Many older people have taken fiber replacements for years on faith thanks to effective advertising. Although this is good for some, as described above, for others extra fiber can be poison. Extra fiber is medicinal if the problem is a fiber deficiency. However, if the problem is poor intestinal movement and/or inadequate water intake, extra fiber can worsen the situation. Many elderly and dying patients take in little water orally. When psyllium and other fiber products are taken with inadequate water, they turn into something like half-dried oatmeal or partially dried cement. This is difficult for the intestine to move. Sometimes large volumes of stool build up and inhibit intestinal movement. The colon dilates and, in effect, goes "on strike." Large, soft impactions can result. Such impactions also frequently occur if the dominant problem is poor bowel motility (see below). Fiber helps with constipation only if the gut is able to respond by pushing it along. Otherwise, fiber may worsen an already bad situation.

Palliative Care Note

Increased fiber intake is relatively contraindicated in the presence of colonic dysmotility and dehydration.

Water

We cannot excrete solid waste without some water. A delicate balance is required; excessive stool water results in diarrhea, and inadequate water results in dry, difficult-to-pass stools. Stool water content depends on how much water we drink, our general hydration status, how much water is secreted and absorbed by the intestine, how fast stool moves through the intestinal tract, and, ultimately, how much water is *retained* in the stool. Manipulating any of these factors can affect stool water. The easiest factor to manipulate is how much water is retained in the stool.

Water is absorbed and secreted into the intestine much more dynamically than most people realize. If certain nonabsorbable or poorly absorbed molecules are present in the intestine, water absorption becomes limited. This is because absorption of water without these molecules would leave a hypertonic solution in the intestine, which is not physiologically possible. (Note: the fiber and solid waste, while making the major contribution to stool volume, chemically has little effect on how concentrated the liquid component of stool is.) Intestinal water can be absorbed only to the extent it leaves a solution behind that is not more concentrated than body water. We can use this property to hold on to water if we need to do so.

Sorbitol and lactulose are concentrated, unabsorbable sugar solutions. Therefore, they are excreted in the stool. These solutions are concentrated, so they must be diluted in the body in order to keep intestinal fluid concentration the same as that of the body. This is accomplished either through "holding on" to water already in the intestine or by moving water from the body into the intestine. The net result is the same: more water in the stool. Lactulose differs from sorbitol in that lactulose is broken into smaller molecules in the large intestine. These smaller, more acidic components make it harder to absorb nitrogenous compounds that may worsen hepatic encephalopathy. Thus, only lactulose should be used if the goal is the treatment of hepatic encephalopathy. In terms of treating constipation, lactulose and sorbitol work in very similar ways. Dosing of these sugars is easily individualized. Although usually given in multiples of 30 ccs, great flexibility in dosing is possible. Many patients, especially the dying, have difficulty tolerating them because of their sickly-sweet taste. Mixing them with juices, especially apple juice, may make them more palatable.

Magnesium salts such as milk of magnesia and magnesium citrate work in a similar fashion to the above agents. They are concentrated solutions that, in effect, "hold onto" water. The main difference is that they are somewhat absorbable. This is usually a problem only for patients who have significant renal failure. As magnesium is excreted by the kidney, renal failure can result in the development of toxic levels, and thus magnesium salts are contraindicated in renal failure. Milk of magnesia is usually given at night in anticipation of an effect by morning. Magnesium citrate comes as a "sparkling laxative." One-half to one bottle is usually given.

Isotonic solutions such as GoLYTELY also contain difficult-to-absorb salts. In contrast to the above agents, they are given in a more dilute form. Thus, significant volumes may have to be drunk or enterally administered in order to produce an effect. The advantage is that they do not draw water from the body. The relatively large volumes required (compared to the 30 ccs commonly given of the agents noted above) may be difficult for some patients, especially the dying, to tolerate.

Phosphate salt enemas similarly contain concentrated, poorly absorbed salts. Such enemas are useful in actively constipated patients who have hard stool in the rectum. Care should be used in patients with congestive heart failure, renal failure, and others who are salt intolerant, especially if used in high enemas, as salt absorption is increased. Excessive use (daily, for example) may cause damage to the rectum.

About high enemas

Refractory impactions proximal to the rectal vault may require treatment with a high enema. There is probably more art than science to the use of such enemas. A variety of fluids may be infused—mineral oil, lubricants, or water. Soapsuds enemas should not be used, as they can irritate colonic mucosa. There is no need to use sterile water or saline. Large water or saline infusions can be problematic in patients who have tenuous fluid balances, such as patients with congestive heart failure.

Movement

There is no M in a BM if there is no *movement* of the bowel. Intestinal movement is complex. The normal gut responds to a variety of stimuli with contractions intended to move contents along. The intestinal volume of water and solid waste leads to gut dilatation and reactive contraction. However, the ability of the intestine to contract lessens if the gut is overly dilated. Imagine trying to squeeze a very large accordion. If your arms are maximally spread apart, the power of your squeeze is weakened. (Similarly, if your hands are very close together, your squeeze is weakened.) Maximum power and ability to squeeze occur at intermediate volumes, and so it is with the intestine. Very small volumes result in little squeeze (and subsequent constipation). Very large volumes, as occurs with impaction, also weaken the ability of the bowel to move.

The gut also responds to signals transmitted by nerves and to direct stimulation of the intestinal lining. As an example of nervous stimulation of the gut, the gastrocolic reflex results in colonic movement due to dilatation of the stomach. Large boluses of food, therefore, stimulate bowel movements. In contrast, small volumes, such as with continuous tube feeding, do not.

Various substances can stimulate the gut and thus cause contractions. Most cathartic medications, such as bisacodyl (Dulcolax), work in this way by directly stimulating the myenteric plexus (nerves in the wall of the intestine). Strong cathartics given either rectally or orally can be helpful if a strong, definitive contraction is desired. These drugs may be useful in trying to clear a constipated stool. Such drugs are best used intermittently, as excessive use may result in a refractory bowel (the bowel goes "on strike"). Other agents, especially senna, may provide a gentler stimulus around the clock, thus counteracting round-the-clock bowel-slowing drugs, such as opioids. Senna is usually started as one to two tablets (187 mg each) qhs and can be advanced to four tablets BID.

A variety of drugs result in intestinal slowing, such as anticholinergic drugs and opioids. Patients taking such drugs should have their medications reviewed to determine if a reduction in dose or elimination of the drug is possible. My experience has been that a fair dose–constipation response exists for anticholinergic drugs. That is, lowering the dose lessens the constipating effect. This seems less true of opioids. Patients on very high doses of opioids may have only slightly more constipation than those on lower doses. Thus, rarely is constipation a reason to reduce the opioid dose if opioids are otherwise indicated. There is evidence that patients on fentanyl experience less constipation than do those on comparable oral opioids.[26–28]

Lubrication

Various agents commonly called stool softeners enhance bowel movements by decreasing friction between the stool and the intestinal wall and rectum by lubricating the stool. Stool is thus easier to pass. These agents minimally soften already hardened stool, but when given orally they may help to prevent hardened stools. Patients who have hemorrhoids, rectal fissures, and other anorectal pathology may become constipated because of pain on the passage of stool. Maintaining a softer, looser stool may help, as does avoidance of foods that may give rise to irritating residua, such as peanuts. Lubricants, as described below, may also be of assistance.

Dioctyl sodium sulfosuccinate (DSS; Colace) decreases surface tension on stool, much like soap. By itself it is usually inadequate in treating opioid-related constipation. DSS is usually given once or twice a day in pill form. Although a liquid form of DSS is available, it should be given only via NG or PEG tubes, not orally, as it tastes like concentrated soap. Although perhaps the most commonly ordered laxative by physicians, the evidence base for the use of DSS is weak.[29]

Mineral oil may be given in enema form and may help to provide lubrication for a previously hard, difficult-to-pass stool. Mineral oil should *not* be given orally, as it may interfere with fat-soluble vitamin absorption and because aspiration may cause pneumonitis.

Glycerin in either stick form or as an enema may similarly lubricate stool and ease passage. It also may increase rectal water by causing rectal water secretion and may stimulate a bowel movement through mechanical rectal stimulation.

While the principles described above should be helpful in reestablishing as normal an intestinal balance as is possible, there is no substitute for frequent evaluation and reevaluation. Patients, family members, and nurses who are most intimately involved in bowel care should generally be given wide latitude in adjusting constipation medications. While some physician oversight may be necessary, excessive control by physicians often results in poorly managed care. If educated, most patients, families, and nurses should be able to adjust medications appropriately on their own.

Bowel Obstruction*

Excellent palliation of bowel obstruction requires experience and skill. Bowel obstruction is one of the most difficult processes to palliate, yet recent advances in understanding and new therapeutic approaches allow us to do a much better job than was possible only a few years ago.[30] That problems like bowel obstruction exist is a compelling reason for why we need palliative care specialists and for why home hospice is not always enough. I have found it very difficult to get bowel obstruction under control when initiating therapy in the home. However, when I can adjust medications on an inpatient unit, I often get people on a regimen that can be administered in home hospice, as happened in the case of Mr. A mentioned at the beginning of this chapter. For those clinicians who believe that palliative care is nothing more than good intentions and a morphine infusion, learning about bowel obstruction can be an eye-opener. Competency requires an understanding of physiology and pharmacology as well as skills in assessment and communication.

Here, I address only the care of malignant bowel obstruction, as this is the type that most commonly arises in palliative care. To what extent this discussion may be applicable to other types of bowel obstruction is unclear. I know of no papers that address the application of the therapies presented here outside of malignant bowel obstruction.

Incidence

Bowel obstruction arises most commonly as a complication of ovarian or colon cancer. In one series 42% of patients with ovarian cancer developed obstruction.[31] Primary presentation of colon cancer with obstruction is usually treated with surgical resection. The incidence of obstruction in colorectal cancer as a late complication is approximately 10%.[32] Other tumors that may give rise to bowel obstruction are gastric, pancreatic, cervical, bladder, endometrial, mesothelial (of peritoneum), carcinoma, and melanoma.

*Based on a presentation to the American Academy of Hospice and Palliative Medicine with copresenter Richard Meyer, M.D., June 1999.

Pathophysiology of Bowel Obstruction

The goal of therapy is to improve quality of life by compensating for the complex and distressing physiologic changes that arise secondary to the obstructive process. This goal is best achieved by normalizing gut function proximal to the obstruction.

The intestinal tract did not evolve to compensate for mechanical bowel obstruction caused by an immobile, fixed lesion such as cancer. The physiologic changes that arise with obstruction would be adaptive to reversible forms of bowel obstruction that may have occurred for our ancient ancestors, but they are maladaptive for patients with cancer. Similarly, kidneys demonstrate a maladaptive response to heart failure. Decreased renal perfusion is sensed as dehydration. Fluid is retained to compensate when, in fact, the patient is drowning. We adjust for this by "overruling" the kidneys, telling them to get rid of salt and water and not hold on to them. The kidneys can be mistaken. What "misunderstanding" arises in bowel obstruction?

Imagine that you have been very hungry. Your tribe finally hunts down a mastodon, and it is time for a feast. You gorge yourself, eating great chunks of meat and causing a temporary obstruction. Your body would respond in the following way.

1. Mechanoreceptors and chemoreceptors would be stimulated by the distention caused by the large build-up of food proximal to the blockage. These receptors would tell your brain to *stop eating*.
2. The intestine proximal to the blockage would begin hypersecreting fluid, trying to flood the system and wash the intestinal contents downstream.
3. Intestinal motility would increase, further trying to push contents downstream and causing cramping.

With luck, you would live to hunt another day. While this approach works well for ingested mastodons, it works poorly for malignant bowel obstruction.

A delicate balance of fluid absorption and secretion from and into the lumen is normally maintained. Studies have demonstrated that with obstruction the balance is shifted strongly in favor of secretion.[33] Increased secretion of fluid results in further intestinal dilatation, cramping, and frank nausea and vomiting. In one small study Huchison measured serotonin levels in women with ovarian cancer with and without bowel obstruction. High levels of urinary 5HIAA, a serotonin metabolite, were found only in obstructed women.[34] This pattern was very similar to the pattern of serotonin elevation found in patients treated with cisplatin. In cisplatin therapy enterochromaffin cells in the intestine secrete serotonin, which binds $5HT_3$ receptors in the gut, thereby stimulating nausea.[35] It is therefore quite possible, but not yet proven, that a similar process occurs in bowel obstruction.

A vicious cycle is entered wherein hypersecretion (associated with cramping in the early stage) is followed by dilatation and vomiting, followed by further secretion and vomiting. Dehydration and electrolyte disturbances quickly result, leading to death (and misery) if an intervention is not made (Fig. 5.2).

Traditional Medical Approaches

Traditional "conservative" management, labeled "drip and suck" therapy by some authors, is an extrapolation from perioperative management for obstruction.[36,37] It certainly makes sense if operating on a vomiting patient with a dilated gut to decompress the gut with an NG tube and restore intravascular volume. However, there is no data that supports this approach as a long-term therapy for malignant bowel obstruction. Indeed, multiple studies have shown dismal outcomes with this approach alone.[38–41] Theoretically, IV hydration, in addition to restoring intravascular volume, also increases hydrostatic pressure in the villi and therefore could increase secretion into the lumen, contributing to the vicious cycle. Mr. A. was initially treated with a traditional drip and suck approach, which still seems to be the dominant approach used in medical care.

Early Palliative Approaches

Early palliative approaches stressed symptomatic relief. It was assumed that the gut was nonfunctional, and therefore no attempt was made to normalize function. Indeed, symptomatic relief, in effect, put the gut to sleep. Anticholinergic drugs, such as hyoscine, both decreased secretion into the gut and decreased

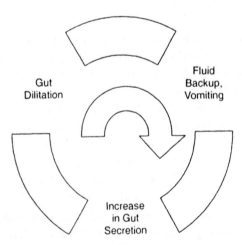

Figure 5.2. Pathophysiology of bowel obstruction—a vicious cycle.

motility, thereby alleviating cramping.[32,42] Opioids were also stressed, both to reduce motility and treat pain directly. These approaches are still used when normalization of gut function is impossible, as it often is in very proximal gut obstruction.

Steroids have been used in the hope of relieving obstruction by reducing swelling around obstructing growths, although their efficacy in this regard is debatable. Bowel obstruction is a very dynamic process, frequently reverting from total to partial obstruction and back in as many as 50% of cases. Only one controlled study of the use of steroids in bowel obstruction has been done. It showed no evidence that steroids were helpful in reducing the degree of obstruction. A major problem in this study was the very high rate of spontaneous conversion from total to partial obstruction.[43] Steroids may nevertheless be useful in bowel obstruction by decreasing bowel and peritoneal inflammation and by acting as appetite stimulants.

Recent Approaches

Recent approaches have tried to normalize gut function to the extent possible in addition to palliating symptoms directly. In practice, the ability to normalize and use the proximal gut is highly dependent on the level of obstruction. Many cases of malignant obstruction that are appropriate for nonsurgical, palliative approaches have multiple sites of obstruction, most frequently in the jejunum or ileum.[44] It is not uncommon to have many feet of potentially functional intestine proximal to the rate-limiting site of obstruction. Very proximal obstructions prohibits normalization. However, very proximal and very distal obstructions may be amenable to stent placement that results in significant palliation by forcing open the gut lumen using an expandable wire mesh stent.[45,46]

Octreotide

The most important drug in the therapy of bowel obstruction is octreotide. An analogue of the hormone somatostatin, it significantly reduces secretion into the gut. In one study by Mangili, 13 patients with ovarian cancer–related obstruction had NG aspirate volumes measured. Mean drainage decreased from 1687 ml/day to < 50 ml/day.[47] Octreotide is generally well tolerated. It appears to have minimal effects on motility. Doses range from 100 mcg BID to 200 mcg TID IV or SC.[48] Octreotide can result in significant improvements in nausea and vomiting.[49] However, because this appears to be due to decreased secretion of fluid into the gut, it usually takes 24 to 48 hours for this effect to become apparent. A recent randomized controlled trial that compared octreotide treatment to scopolamine butylbromide (an anticholinergic agent unavailable in the United States) demonstrated that octreotide was superior in reducing intestinal secretions.[50] A new long-acting depo version of octreotide has been developed. I am unfamiliar with any studies that used it in bowel obstruction. In theory, one injection can last up to a month. However, it is very expensive.

Promotility agents

Promotility agents can be used if cramping is not present and if the intention is to normalize and use the proximal gut. Traditionally, clinicians have believed that promotility agents are contraindicated in bowel obstruction because increased motility could worsen cramping and theoretically result in gut perforation. However, reports of the beneficial effects of promotility drugs are beginning to appear in the literature.[36,51] There are, to my reading, no data to substantiate the concern about inducing perforation. I am unaware of a single case report that associates bowel perforation or rupture with promotility drug use. Metoclopramide is the drug of choice for this purpose. Metoclopramide works by binding $5HT_4$ receptors and releasing acetylcholine, which in turn binds cholinergic receptors and results in increased motility. Understanding this is important, as concomitant use of drugs with anticholinergic effects, such as scopolamine, promethazine, or amitriptyline, may antagonize this action and reduce efficacy. Dosing is usually begun at 10 mg TID AC PO and gradually increased. Care should be used with metoclopramide in the presence of renal failure, as it is renally excreted, and in patients with Parkinson's disease because of dopamine receptor blockade. For large bowel obstruction a combination of metoclopramide with a large bowel stimulant, such as senna, will probably have to suffice until new motility agents are identified. Experts in the field have warned that promotility drugs should not be used in complete bowel obstruction, although the evidence base for this seems weak, as mentioned above.[30] In practice it is not always easy to distinguish total from partial obstruction. Frequently, obstruction progresses from partial to total and back again, making the advice not to use promotility drugs in total obstruction easier to give in principle than to follow in practice.

Direct antiemetics

If cramping is present or if the intent is to rest the bowel, as with patients no longer capable of eating or drinking, anticholinergic and antihistaminic antiemetics such as promethazine may be used. (See section on nausea.) Glycopyrrolate, a more locally acting anticholinergic drug, can be given orally or parenterally. It can reduce cramping, intestinal secretion, and nausea.

If the goal is to normalize gut function, anticholinergic agents should be avoided, because they both inhibit motility and block the use of metoclopramide. Many experts use haloperidol as a first-line agent in part because it does not affect motility. However, a pharmacologic rationale for this is lacking, as it is unclear that dopamine receptors are significantly involved in the pathophysiology of obstructive nausea. I suspect $5HT_3$ antagonists, such as ondansetron, may be the agents of choice, based on the limited data presented above suggesting $5HT_3$-mediated nausea and the fact that they have limited effects on motility.[52] They are expensive, however, and the evidence base for this practice has not been established.

Other interventions include:

NG/venting gastrostomies. Although NG tube placement is a bad approach, I believe, for long-term management in most cases, it can be very helpful for initial gut decompression. I often keep NG tubes in place during initiation of octreotide. Venting gastrostomies have been used, much like PEG tubes for feeding, as a long-term alternative to NG tubes for decompression. Although certainly less uncomfortable than NG tubes, there is minimal evidence that they result in less nausea or distention. No studies have compared venting gastrostomies to long-term octreotide therapy. A consensus panel of the European Association of Palliative Care recommended that venting gastrostomies be used only if medications fail to control nausea.[30]

Simethicone. I have given patients who are not acutely vomiting simethicone in order to encourage burping of stomach and intestinal gas. Although not yet documented as efficacious in the literature, in my experience this is nontoxic and simply makes sense. One cause of intestinal dilatation is intestinal gas (largely nitrogen) that cannot be disposed of "the old-fashioned way" via flatus. Studies have shown that the vast majority of gas seen on an abdominal X-ray is swallowed.[33] To the extent dilatation directly contributes to the vicious cycle described above, it makes sense to do everything possible to minimize dilatation, including encouraging burping. The usual dose is 80 mg BID to TID.

Low-fiber diet. Most patients with bowel obstruction who are able to eat should be on a low-fiber diet. This is essential if they are trying to eat with a total obstruction (as is, in fact, sometimes possible). Patients with complete obstruction who do eat often vomit or regurgitate every few days. Although this is not pleasant, it appears to be more pleasant than dying with an NG tube.

Opioids. Opioids are very effective in dealing with the cramping of bowel obstruction and are usually needed for pain management associated with advanced malignant disease. However, they can have undesirable effects on motility if one is trying to normalize gut function. As a general rule, pain management trumps motility management. That is, if a patient needs an opioid for pain, give it. As previously discussed, the fentanyl patch may have a lesser effect on GI motility than do other agents. It is often preferred, as well, because the oral route is generally unreliable in bowel obstruction.

Psychosocial support. So far, the emphasis has been on physiology. Bowel obstruction also requires psychosocial support. Patients with distal obstruction often become distended, which alters body image and can be distressing. While most patients hate NG tubes, they can also become dependent on them and may resist suggestions to discontinue them. This may be because when they were initially placed they did provide relief. Such patients also probably fear possible tube replacement. Tubes although discouraged as long-term therapy, may also represent medical caring, and thus patients and families may view suggestions to discontinue them as potential abandonment. The rationale for discontinuation of any therapy, as discussed elsewhere, must be carefully explained. As discussed later in the section on cachexia and anorexia, the inability to eat or drink normally causes an intense grief reaction in patients and families. Adjusting the diet, usually to low-fiber liquid-based formulations, may allow nurturing to continue even in the presence of complete bowel obstruction.

What Does Success Look Like in the Treatment of Bowel Obstruction?

In my experience most patients with bowel obstruction can have NG tubes and IVs discontinued. In some very proximal cases I have continued both if medications do not adequately control secretions. The symptoms of pain, bloating, nausea, and vomiting should be amendable to palliation in virtually all cases. In the most rewarding cases I have treated, such as Mr. A., patients with total distal bowel obstruction who probably would have died within days with traditional drip and suck therapy have been able to resume eating, improve their functional status, and be discharged to home, living for weeks to a few months postobstruction. Although the treatment of bowel obstruction is difficult, it can be very rewarding. Controlled trials have not been performed on all the interventions suggested above. I hope they will be done in the near future in hopes of furthering our understanding and expanding our treatment options.

Mouth Care

Symptoms related to the mouth are prevalent at the end of life and are often overlooked by clinicians.[53,54] The mouth may become too dry (xerostomia), or patients may be troubled by excess salivary production (sialorrhea). They may experience drooling or choking if they are unable to handle the complex steps involved in swallowing saliva. They are also prone to a variety of infections—candidiasis, viral infections (especially herpes in immuno-suppressed patients), and some bacterial infections.

Good mouth care is important to maintain quality of life. Speaking, the pleasure of eating, and the normal handling of saliva are taken for granted by most of us. It may be difficult to imagine the impact mouth disorders have on patients. As the mouth is largely hidden, the patient, family, and caregivers may not recognize problems when they occur. As an exercise, the reader is encouraged to consciously hold his or her mouth open for several minutes. Saliva will begin to pool about the lower teeth. At the same time the tongue will dry. Drooling eventually will occur. Suddenly, what we have taken for granted, swallowing spit, becomes precious.

Palliative Care Note

In end-of-life care examination and reexamination of the mouth is one of the most important tasks.

Xerostomia (Dry Mouth)

Common causes of xerostomia are

- medications (anticholinergic agents, opioids to a lesser degree, clonidine)
- dehydration
- mouth breathing
- surgery or radiotherapy to the mouth
- infections of the mouth

Dry mouth is very prevalent and troublesome. As this list suggests, treatable causes are common. Taking patients off of unnecessary anticholinergic medications, for example, can be of great help. Other causes, such as dehydration, radiation-related xerostomia, and mouth breathing may be harder to address directly.

The relationships between dehydration, thirst, and dry mouth are complex and frequently misunderstood. They are discussed in more detail in the chapter 6. While systemic dehydration undoubtedly contributes to decreased saliva production, rehydration with IV fluids, for example, does not necessarily correct the problem and may be associated with undesired side effects, such as worsening respiratory secretions. Side effects of medications, especially anticholinergic agents and opioids, and mouth breathing may significantly contribute to this symptom.

Treatment

For most patients simple therapies such as frequent sips of water, ice chips, and swabbing of the mouth with a moist sponge on a stick are usually sufficient.[55] Glycerin swabs have been discouraged by some because they are hyperosmolar and thus further dry the tongue and mucosa by drawing fluid from tissue. Lemon drops or other sour candies can stimulate saliva, and the sour flavor is often preferred by dying patients. A variety of artificial salivas, usually based on methyl-cellulose, can also be prescribed and may keep the mouth moist longer than does pure water. Pilocarpine, a cholinergic agonist, has been shown to significantly increase saliva production, even in radiation-induced xerostomia. Pilocarpine is usually started at 2.5 mg TID with studies suggesting 5 mg TID as the dose which is most efficacious with minimal side effects.[53] Side effects relate to cholinergic stimulation, including sweating, cramping, bradycardia, and bronchospasm in those prone to wheezing. Thus, this drug is contraindicated in patients who have bradycardia or bronchospasm.

Difficulty Handling Saliva, Drooling, and Sialorrhea

In rare cases patients may produce excess saliva. More commonly, they have difficulty handling normally produced saliva because of alterations in mouth anatomy or because of impaired neurologic control of the swallowing reflex. The latter, often manifested by drooling, is the more common. Drooling carries a great social stigma and can be very disturbing to patients and families. Patients with Parkinson's disease, amyotrophic lateral sclerosis, cerebral vascular accidents, dementia, and developmental disorders are prone to this. Patients in the very advanced stages of dying may also experience difficulties as they loose their swallowing and cough reflexes.

Usually, the underlying cause is untreatable. However, anticholinergic agents can be of some help in decreasing salivary flow. Care should be taken in using systemically absorbable agents, as they can produce troubling side effects. In addition, for some patients the dry mouth that results from medication may be as troubling as the earlier drooling. Studies in developmentally delayed children and more recent studies of adults who drool suggest that glycopyrrolate may be effective in decreasing salivary production with little, if any, systemic toxicity.[56,57] Glycopyrrolate is an anticholinergic agent that is poorly absorbed from the GI tract and that minimally crosses the blood–brain barrier if given systemically (as it often is in anesthesia). I have had some success with this agent. Tablets of 1 mg can be dissolved in a small amount of water and held in the mouth (or swabbed onto mucosa if unable to be held) and then spit out. This is usually given BID or TID. If swallowed, glycopyrrolate will have a strong local anticholinergic effect on the GI tract and decrease motility and secretion into the gut. This will worsen constipation or treat diarrhea but decrease the systemic effect, as only 5% of the drug is absorbed. As the goal of therapy is to reduce the production of saliva, *not* to dry the mouth completely, the mouth should be moistened with artificial saliva if secondary xerostomia results.

Candidiasis

Candidal infections of the mouth occur frequently, especially in patients who are on steroids and in diabetics. Thrush is relatively easy to recognize. White cottage cheese–like plaques are found, often associated with tenderness, dysphagia, and altered taste (dysgeusia). More difficult to recognize are the atrophic forms, both acute and chronic. Acute atrophic candidiasis usually presents as a reddened tongue with depapillation, which is also associated with dysgeusia. It is my impression that this form may be more common in patients with xerostomia, as inadequate moisture exists to create classic thrush. Vitamin deficiencies, poor nutrition, and xerostomia itself may all create a similar picture, making definitive diagnosis difficult on exam alone. Chronic atrophic candidiasis is similar to acute (reddened mucosa, especially in the area where upper dentures are in contact with the palate) and is most common in elderly patients with dentures. It is often associated with angular cheilitis, which is painful.

A variety of antifungals can be employed in therapy. Nystatin suspension is often well tolerated, as it is a liquid. Because efficacy relates to drug contact time with the mucosa, some caregivers make small "popsicles" with toothpicks for patients to suck on. Some strains of candida are resistant and may respond better to other agents. Mycelex troches are typically given five times a day, although less frequent administration can be given to the dying. Patients with significant xerostomia may have trouble dissolving troches. Systemic agents, such as fluconazole are rarely required and are expensive. Fluconazole may be indicated for resistant strains and when candida is suspected beyond the GI tract, such as when a patient has new-onset hoarseness with a sore throat in association with oral candida (often indicative of laryngeal involvement).

Viral and Bacterial Infections

Immuno-suppressed patients are at a higher risk for both viral (predominantly herpes simplex) and bacterial infections. Herpes infections should be suspected when such patients have new-onset pain or odynophagia (common with esophageal herpes); it is best treated with acyclovir. Patients with xerostomia appear to be at higher risk of bacterial parotitis and present with the sudden onset of a firm, warm, painful swelling under the angle of the jaw. They may be susceptible because of decreased salivary flow from the parotid gland. Broad-spectrum treatment with an antibiotic such as Augmentin is usually effective.

Mouth and Esophageal Pain

Pain in the mouth and esophagus can result from a variety of causes, including infections, radiation, and chemotherapy, among others. Good oral hygiene is important for all causes. A variety of concoctions have been developed specifically to treat this pain. Most have not been rigorously studied or compared for efficacy. Lidocaine and benzocaine sprays can be useful on oral lesions. For esophageal pain, viscous lidocaine 2% is commonly used. Traditionally, 5–15 ccs are given every four hours. However, in my experience the duration of efficacy is considerably shorter than this. Duration of analgesia appears to be closely linked to duration of exposure of the mucosa to the anesthetic. A variety of "thickening agents" have been used to try to prolong this action—milk of magnesia, for example—although I am unaware of formal studies to evaluate the degree to which duration of action might be prolonged.

Dyspnea

Dyspnea is a common and distressing symptom.[58] In the National Hospice Study 70% of patients experienced dyspnea in the final six weeks of life.[59] Bruera and colleagues found that 55% of 135 patients with advanced cancer experienced moderate dyspnea.[60] Not surprisingly, lung involvement with cancer correlated strongly with dyspnea in this study (as did anxiety and maximal inspiratory pressure). Chronic obstructive pulmonary disease (COPD), congestive heart failure, and fluid build-up in renal failure can also cause dyspnea. Because of the high prevalence of this symptom and the severity of suffering that can be associated with it, clinicians need to become familiar with available methods for the alleviation of dyspnea.[61] Dyspnea is also not rare in a variety of nonterminal illnesses. Standard medical therapies often address this symptom and are "palliative" in that treatment is not curative of the underlying disease. Examples include most treatments for COPD and congestive heart failure. Therapies effective in standard treatment may also be effective at the end of life. However, certain important distinctions need to be made.

In standard medical therapy treatment for dyspnea is directed toward both alleviating dyspnea and prolonging the patient's life. This is entirely appropriate for many patients. An example would be the administration of ACE (angiotensin converting enzyme) inhibitors for congestive heart failure. These medications both relieve dyspnea by decreasing pulmonary edema through afterload reduction and can prolong life. ACE inhibitors may also be used in patients with congestive heart failure whose primary treatment goal is comfort. However, the life-prolonging aspect of the therapy should be carefully considered. For some, such modest life-prolonging effects may be entirely acceptable, even desirable. For others, at a certain stage even modest life-prolonging "side effects" of ACE inhibitors may be considered a burden. Alternate methods of alleviating dyspnea that do not have life-prolonging side effects should be considered.

Traditional medical therapy for dyspnea focuses almost exclusively on altering physiology in the lungs and elsewhere (heart and kidneys). Bronchodilators open small airways. Diuretics reduce fluid build-up. Antibiotics kill organisms that disrupt lung function. Rarely is the *sensation* or other psychic aspects of the experience directly addressed. As discussed in Chapter 3, in palliative care the totality of the patient's experience that results in suffering should be addressed.

Pathophysiology of Dyspnea

Dyspnea is the experience of shortness of breath. It may or may not be associated with suffering. A runner in a race may be severely dyspneic and yet be enjoying life. A dyspneic patient dying with lung cancer with very similar physiologic parameters may be suffering greatly, as the meaning and context of the dyspnea are entirely different.

Respiration as a bodily function is virtually unique in the degree to which it is under both reflexive and volitional control. The survival advantage of such a control is obvious. We continue to breath when deeply asleep (or in a coma), and yet we can hold our breath, if need be, to escape through smoke or water. Perhaps because of this, the linkage between psychological states and breathing is tighter and more complex than it is for other physical symptoms. Dyspnea is often associated with panic and anxiety; panic may present as dyspnea, and dyspnea may induce panic.

My education about dyspnea, brief as it was in medical school, stressed the importance of blood gases. I learned that CO_2 build-up and oxygen deprivation were the critical factors that result in dyspnea. Although undoubtedly important in keeping the body alive, their importance in the experience of dyspnea has been exaggerated. If an oxygen saturation monitor is attached to a dyspneic runner at the end of a race, it will register normal. This reveals an important clinical pearl: oxygen saturation is insensitive in identifying patients with dyspnea. That is, one cannot rely on the oxygen saturation to tell who is dyspneic. Patients can be very dyspneic with normal saturations. Of course, patients with low oxygen saturations (below 90%) are far more likely to be dyspneic than are patients with normal saturations. However, oxygen saturation also lacks specificity as a predictor of dyspnea; many patients with low oxygen saturations (for example, patients with chronic lung disease or those who live at high altitude) will not be dyspneic, especially at rest. Studies have suggested that hypoxia correlates best with exertional dyspnea and poor exercise tolerance. Conversely, oxygen therapy has been shown to be a most helpful method to relieve exertional dyspnea and improve exercise tolerance. Studies have been mixed in testing the relief of rest dyspnea associated with hypoxia with oxygen therapy.[62,63] Oxygen levels are excellent indicators of changing pulmonary physiology. The implications of the lack of sensitivity and specificity of oxygen saturation in identifying dyspnea are profound. As with pain, we lack a "scanner" for dyspnea that can reliably identify who is short of breath. We have no choice but to *ask* if dyspnea is present, or at least look for signs of distress that might suggest dyspnea, such as rapid respirations or a look of panic. In fact, the oxygen saturation meter can *cause* dyspnea by inducing panic and fear in patients, family, and clinicians as the saturation number falls (often accompanied by an ominously lower-pitched beeping tone).

Palliative Care Note

Oxygen saturation cannot be depended upon to identify dyspnea. Patient report or signs of agitation or anxiety are the best means of identifying dyspnea.

Elevations in carbon dioxide levels appear to stimulate dyspnea more than do low oxygen levels. Elevated partial pressure of arterial carbon dioxide (Pa_{CO2}) levels have been found to be an independent stimulus of dyspnea.[64] However, increased respiratory drive does not necessarily result in dyspnea if it occurs unimpeded. Patients with certain forms of increased respiratory drive, such as diabetic ketoacidosis and pregnancy, may not experience dyspnea. *What does cause dyspnea is an imbalance between the perceived need to breathe and the perceived ability to breathe.* Elevated Pa_{CO2} levels may be one among a number of factors that contribute to the brain's perception of a need to breathe.

Palliative Care Note

Dyspnea results when there is an imbalance between the perceived *need* to breathe and the perceived *ability* to breathe.

Recent studies have suggested that the body's ability to determine whether breathing is occurring normally relies on considerably more than high CO_2 levels or low oxygen levels.[64] Nerves in the nose sense the passage of air. Stretch receptors in and about the lungs signal expansion and contraction of the lungs. Thoracic muscles and ribs signal that they are moving, a good sign breathing is occurring normally. These nerves tell the brain "all is well" and allow respirations to continue automatically and largely unconsciously in the nondyspneic person. The brain senses no imbalance between the ability to breathe and the need to breathe. If there is a sudden cessation of airflow or respiratory muscle movement, as measured by these nerves, the brain quickly goes into alarm mode—before any measurable change in blood gases occurs.

Imagine you are being held one foot below water. Go ahead—hold your breath. Note how quickly there is a desire to breathe. You can suppress this need for a while, although it will build rapidly. (Your oxygen saturation may fall slightly and your CO_2 saturation may rise slightly by the time you must breathe, contributing a bit to the need to breathe.) If you were truly underwater, you would panic almost immediately. This psychological state would result in a severe imbalance between the perceived need to breathe and the perceived ability to breathe. You would desperately struggle to get to the surface. When you finally breathe again, notice how quickly your dyspnea is relieved. Do you really believe it was because your blood gases were so quickly normalized?

Patients more commonly are dyspneic *while* breathing. What is happening here? The perception of respiratory fatigue is a key component. Although our understanding of both peripheral and central receptor involvement in fatigue is poor, it is clear that the brain is able to sense fatigue, much as you can sense any overworked muscle. However, unlike wobbly leg muscles that signal you to stop running, tired thoracic muscles must continue to work in an attempt to meet a perceived need to breathe. The brain senses a mismatch: the need to breathe continues, but the ability of the body to meet that need with tired muscles is in doubt. Dyspnea is a wake-up call to this mismatch.

Short of altering lung physiology, how can this mismatch be addressed? Decreasing the perceived need through energy conservation can help. Patients with emphysema, who have minimal thoracic expansion, may ventilate adequately but receive a signal from the thoracic muscles that they are not moving enough, much as in the underwater example above. A number of studies have demonstrated that fooling these muscles by activating vibrating devices during inspiration can lessen dyspnea.[65–67] The perception that the body is not able to meet this need can also be addressed by inhibiting the perception of muscular fatigue with opioids and other drugs (see below).

As should have been apparent in the breath-holding experiment, perceived need is also intimately connected to the psyche. Perceived need and perceived inability to meet that need can quickly result in panic. Panic, in turn, can stimulate increased ventilatory effort, which can result in more fatigue and increased panic—a vicious cycle. Panic, fear, and anxiety are common affective components of dyspnea. Beyond shear panic, dyspneic patients *think* about what their dyspnea means. Does dyspnea reflect a good run, as it might to a jogger, or impending death? If dyspnea occurs with increasingly mild exertion, the patient is reminded of growing dependence on others. As with other symptoms, patients monitor the trend of their dyspnea—is it getting better or worse? One reason the runner does not suffer from dyspnea is that he or she knows it will end when the running ends. The patient dying of COPD or lung cancer projects into a future wherein dyspnea worsens. These cognitive processes commonly trigger affective responses. In addition to panic, fear, and anxiety, patients may become depressed and angry.

Dyspnea Treatment Principles

Here I address only those therapies not commonly employed in the traditional treatment of dyspnea. Traditional palliative measures focus on altering lung physiology by using beta agonists, diuretics, or tapping pleural effusions. Understanding the physiology of dyspnea as presented above suggests that when altering lung physiology fails, altering the perceived need and perceived ability to meet that need should improve the sensation of dyspnea. Addressing affective and cognitive components of dyspnea should alleviate its psychic components.

Opioids and benzodiazepines are the mainstays of palliative therapy for dyspnea. In choosing between starting an opioid or a benzodiazepine treatment for a dyspneic patient, the patient may give you a hint as to which is likely to be more effective. A patient who complains of hard work breathing but who lacks associated anxiety is more likely to benefit from an opioid. A patient who complains of anxiety associated with breathing is usually better first treated with a benzodiazepine. Having said this, often both are tried to determine which drug class is better for the patient. Prediction based on this rule of thumb is imperfect. Many patients will need both classes of medication and may be able to state clear preferences for "breakthrough" doses for exacerbations of dyspnea.

Opioids

Opioids are very effective in relieving dyspnea, although the exact mechanism is not understood. Contrary to common belief, this effect does not result through inhibition of respiratory drive. Relief from the "work of breathing" is a function of steady-state opioid levels, much like steady-state opioid levels relieve pain. Inhibition of respiratory drive results primarily from rising opioid serum levels. Studies have demonstrated significant relief of dyspnea from opioids without significant effects on ventilation or pCO_2 levels in common therapeutic doses.[68,69] Having said this, patients with dyspnea are fragile. Respiratory drive suppression can occur if serum opioid levels rise rapidly. Thus, when initiating therapy with opioids for dyspnea, one should start with a low dose and raise the dose *slowly* as needed.

Morphine is the best studied of the opioids for relief of dyspnea, although relief has been observed with other agents, such as oxycodone, fentanyl, and methadone. There is no demonstrated advantage of one opioid over another. Generally, a lower dose of opioid is required to relieve dyspnea than is needed to relieve pain.

Nebulized morphine has been used by some to treat dyspnea, although this is not an FDA-approved route of administration in the United States.[70] Mu receptors, to which morphine binds, have been identified in the lung, and it has been theorized that binding of these peripheral receptors may relieve dyspnea at lower serum levels of morphine than when it is given via other routes. Studies have demonstrated that aerosolized morphine is effective in the relief of dyspnea, although no clear advantage of this route has yet been proven other than its rapid onset of action. Few bioavailability studies have been done. From 5% to 100% bioavailability has been reported.[71] I believe it safest to assume 100%

bioavailability, at least with initial dosing. One advantage of the aerosolized route is that peak serum levels occur rapidly—roughly equal to the time it takes to deliver the aerosol. This can be an advantage over oral dosing (peak effect in one hour) and parenteral administration, which may not be feasible in certain settings, such as in the home.

Morphine can cause histamine release, thereby inducing bronchospasm when given by aerosol. (See chapter 4, section on morphine.) It may be wise to give a trial dose under observation and to watch for bronchospasm. It seems advisable to ensure that patients are able to tolerate nonaerosolized morphine with no histamine release before attempting aerosol therapy. There has been some concern that the preservatives for regular IV morphine may trigger bronchospasm, although, to my knowledge, this is only theoretical. Thus, some authors have recommended using preservative-free morphine when using aerosol. I have successfully used injectable (*not oral solution*) morphine in a number of patients with no evidence of adverse effect.

In my practice I have used this route primarily when a patient is already receiving other nebulized medications to which morphine can be added or when rapid, nonparenteral (IV, SC) dosing is desired. Responses appear to be somewhat idiosyncratic. Some patients love it, while others are unimpressed. I recommend starting with a low dose, 2–4 mgs. I have not read of experiences with other opioids administered via this route.

Benzodiazepines

Benzodiazepines are very helpful in relieving panic and anxiety associated with dyspnea, if present, but are not helpful if panic and anxiety are absent.[6] Lorazepam is most commonly used in low doses. Longer-acting benzodiazepines may also be used for chronic dyspnea. This effect also does not appear to be directly related to suppression of respiratory drive. As with opioids, respiratory drive can be suppressed by benzodiazepines if they are escalated rapidly and given in high doses. Thus, rapid escalation of benzodiazepines, especially via the IV route, should be avoided. Start *low* and go *slow*.

Other agents

Identifying an agent that reliably alleviates dyspnea without risk of respiratory drive suppression would be the palliative care equivalent of finding the Holy Grail. So far, efforts have largely failed. It was hoped that local anesthetics, such as lidocaine, would numb stretch receptors and in so doing alleviate dyspnea, but this has not been found to be the case.[72] Further research in this area is needed.

Oxygen may relieve dyspnea, especially when significant hypoxia (O_2 sat <90) is present during exercise. In addition, oxygen may relieve dyspnea via other mechanisms. Airway resistance may be decreased when oxygen is administered,

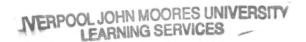

thereby reducing the work of breathing.[73] The flow of gas over the nasal mucosa may itself provide a dampening effect on the perception of dyspnea. Liss and Grant randomized patients to receive oxygen or air via nasal prongs at 2 or 4 liters. Dyspnea was equally relieved by both therapies. Dyspnea increased when the nasal mucosa was anesthetized.[74] This study can be criticized for having treated patients with relatively high mean pO_2 levels (67 mm Hg) and for having treated only rest dyspnea.[62] In a later double-blind cross-over study by Bruera and colleagues, 14 hypoxemic cancer patients were randomized to receive oxygen or air by mask. Twelve of fourteen patients consistently preferred oxygen. Visual analogue scale reports of dyspnea were significantly less on oxygen compared to air.[63] While oxygen therefore may be very helpful, patients who are confused or distressed may not tolerate oxygen administration, especially via mask, as masks may be constricting. Such patients often respond better to a gentle fan or cool breeze.

Cachexia, Anorexia, and Asthenia

Cachexia

Cachexia (tissue wasting), anorexia (lack of appetite), and asthenia (weakness) frequently arise in palliative care and often overlap. The pathophysiologic processes involved are complex and may vary from one disease process to another. Cancer-associated cachexia has been most researched. Many other diseases associated with wasting are less well studied. One thing is clear—it is overly simplistic to extrapolate from starvation to the wasting syndromes of chronic illnesses. It is also dangerous to extrapolate from one disease to another, as different diseases may have very different pathophysiologies.

Because cancer-related cachexia is relatively well understood (compared to other diseases), I focus on this. The concern of many patients, families, and clinicians is that patients who are losing weight and energy in advanced stages of cancer are, in fact, starving to death. In most cases the process is very different from starvation.[75] It may sound strange, but humans were designed for starvation. That is, we evolved over millennia to survive periodic episodes of starvation. True starvation responses are geared for enhanced survival. In starvation hunger is initially dramatically increased; later it fades. Initial gut cramping that is experienced with starvation milks the intestine, which prevents bacterial overgrowth. The body shifts its metabolism to a slow, catabolic mode, which minimizes energy expenditure while preserving critically needed lean body mass until no other calories remain to be burned. Upon refeeding, assuming this is not done too quickly, appetite grows, the body shifts to an anabolic metabolic mode, and lean body mass is soon replenished.[76] Refeeding dramatically increases the chance of survival.

The situation could not be more different in cancer-related cachexia. (Here, I am assuming that reversible causes of not eating or gaining weight, such as dysphagia, depression, nausea, and malabsorption have been addressed.) Appetite is lost early in the process. Gut cramping tends not to occur. The body becomes catabolic, but in a dysfunctional way. Total body energy expenditures may be increased, normal, or decreased. Lean body mass is not necessarily preserved. Refeeding either by tube feeding or total parenteral nutrition (TPN) in advanced disease does not replenish lean body mass, as it would in starvation. Patients' functional statuses do not improve, nor is survival improved. The details of the biochemical changes associated with cancer-related cachexia are beginning to be understood. It appears that a variety of tumor-associated cytokines, such as tumor necrosis factor (TNF), IL-1, IL-6, and LIF, are involved in this pathologic response.[77-79] It seems likely that future therapy to modulate or block these mediators will alter the currently inexorable course associated with cancer-related cachexia.

Although the details of how cancer-related cachexia differs from starvation are probably beyond the understanding of most patients and families, we often need to summarize this information for them. Many will not accept that cancer-related cachexia is not starvation. For most people it seems obvious that if a patient is not eating and is losing weight, he or she needs to be re-fed. If the patient is unable to take food naturally, one simply needs to override the system and feed artificially. Although similar processes may be involved in cachexia related to other diseases, such as congestive heart failure and dementia (although these and other diseases with associated cachexia are poorly studied), a special cautionary note must be voiced relating to AIDS.[80] Certain patients with AIDS have demonstrated functional improvement and increased lean body mass with artificial feeding, highlighting the fact that real differences exist among different illnesses.[81]

Anorexia

Anorexia (lack of appetite) is prevalent in advanced cancer and in many advanced chronic illnesses.[82] For patients who die over a prolonged period of time, anorexia usually occurs in the last weeks to days of life. In the terminal phase lack of appetite is often the first in a series of normal losses. (See Chapter 11 on the final 48 hours.) In earlier phases care must be taken to rule out reversible causes of anorexia, such as mouth infections, dysgeusia (abnormal taste) related to chemotherapy or zinc deficiency, pain, nausea, and, depression.[83]

What is the suffering in the loss of appetite? Loss of appetite represents the loss of a pleasurable experience, eating. This loss of a primordial pleasure usually results in a grief reaction. Families grieve the loss of the ability to nurture, and patients grieve the loss of being nurtured in this most basic of ways. Understanding the nature of these losses helps caregivers to work with patients and families beyond simply trying to improve appetite. Families may need to be coached in how to nurture without measuring nurturing in terms of the amount consumed. A favorite ice cream or pudding would likely be more refreshing for the patient than would a three-course meal. Similarly, patients can be encouraged to "indulge" by eating small amounts of favored foods simply for the pleasure of taste.

Appetite stimulants

Cancer and HIV have been most studied in terms of appetite stimulants. Less is known about appetite stimulation in other diseases. A variety of agents have been tried.[84] The best-known are megestrol, dronabinol, and steroids. It is important to separate the effects of these drugs on appetite from their effects on building lean body mass and improving functional status. In cancer, at least, the major effect of all these agents is on appetite. If present at all in cancer, weight gain, especially with megestrol and steroids, reflects either water or fat gain, not a gain in lean body mass.[85,86] In cancer appetite stimulation is just that—appetite stimulation—not a method of overriding cancer-related cachexia. All three agents have been found to be effective in series of patients. Megestrol must be given in high doses, approximately 800 mg a day. It is generally well tolerated. Dronabinol, a tetra hydro cannabinol (THC) derivative, may also be effective. It has been best studied in HIV, in which a placebo-controlled trial demonstrated improved appetite.[87] It may be associated with mental status changes, which may be welcomed or disturbing. Steroids, such as dexamethasone, are effective appetite stimulants. Dexamethasone is also a useful adjuvant in pain management and as an anti-inflammatory. Dexamethasone is most helpful in the terminal phase of illness, the last few weeks to months of life. If used before this stage for appetite stimulation, side effects such as immunosuppression, steroid-related myopathy, and osteoporosis may result in burdens that outweigh the benefits.

At some point even those patients who initially respond to appetite stimulants will lose their appetite. Unless the appetite stimulating medication, such as dexamethasone, is being given for another purpose, there is no medical benefit in continuing such therapy. Patients and families may resist efforts to discontinue therapy out of grief—giving up the medication may mean acknowledging progression of illness and another loss in a series of losses. Careful explanation and attention to the grief reaction that usually accompanies such discontinuation is important.

Asthenia

The most mysterious element of this triad for me is asthenia (lack of energy). Asthenia and its opposite, vigor, are familiar to all of us. Everyday, we hope, we start the day refreshed. By the end of the day we are tired, asthenic, and ready to sleep. Even catching a cold can dramatically influence our energy levels. We become weak and tired for no reason identifiable on a blood test. This is a part of our everyday experience. If a cold or a busy day at work can do that, think what a life-threatening chronic illness and dying can do. Clinicians, despite being very aware of their own periodic asthenia, have largely ignored asthenia in their patients. Where does this weakness come from? In cancer and in many other conditions such as advanced dementia and very old age (>95), asthenia appears to be a major cause of death. This is quite remarkable. Arguably, in chronic illnesses that do not directly destroy vital organs (such as heart, lung, kidney, brain, or liver), asthenia (or the "dwindles" in common vernacular) is *the* leading cause of death, yet we have paid very little attention to it. Most cancers do not metastasize to vital organs such as the heart, and if they do death occurs long before organ failure occurs. They seem to kill in some very poorly understood way by weakening the body such that it succumbs to degenerative processes. In cancer asthenia correlates poorly with tumor mass. I have seen some patients with prostate cancer whose bone scans have shown their entire axial skeleton replaced by tumor yet who maintain good energy levels. Other cancer patients with overtly small tumor burdens take to their beds and inexorably die in a matter of days or weeks. Much of this asthenic effect may relate to tumor-related cytokines, as previously described. Perhaps one day physicians will focus on helping people live *with* their cancers by interfering with these mediators when tumors cannot be eradicated.

Even if we do come up with a cure for cancer, this will inevitably result in more patients who live to very old ages. Many geriatric patients of very advanced age appear to "melt," developing severe cachexia, anorexia, and profound asthenia in the months or years prior to death. We do not understand this pathophysiology well at all.

There are some correctable causes of asthenia that are familiar to most clinicians. Hypothyroidism, anemia, and depression can result in reversible asthenia and should be diagnosed and corrected when possible. Untreated pain, other metabolic abnormalities such as adrenal insufficiency, hypokalemia, and steroid-related myopathy may also manifest as asthenia.

A special note needs to be made about treating anemia as a cause of asthenia. Many patients with anemia respond well to either transfusions or stimulation of red cell production with erythropoietin, both of which increase energy and functional status.[88] However, a point usually comes when patients no longer get the same "bounce" out transfusions that they once did, especially if they are dying of some chronic illness. Their asthenia becomes refractory to such interventions. Patients, families, and even clinicians may have trouble recognizing or acknowledging this change. Getting transfusions then becomes a ritual in which caring is shown. Suggesting that transfusions may no longer be useful for the desired purpose (when treating asthenia) may be hard to accept and may result in grief reactions that must be addressed.

References

1. Hornby, P. J. Central neurocircuitry associated with emesis. Am J Med 2001; 111(suppl 8A): 106S–12S.
2. Mannix, K. Palliation of nausea and vomiting. In: D. Doyle, G. Hanks, et al., eds. *The Oxford Textbook of Palliative Medicine*. 1998, Oxford University Press: New York, pp. 490–8.
3. Rousseau, P. Non-pain symptom management in terminal care. Clin Geriatr Med 1996; 12: 313–6.
4. Hesketh, P. J. et al. Randomized phase II study of the neurokinin 1 receptor antagonist CJ- 11,974 in the control of cisplatin-induced emesis. J Clin Oncol 1999; 17(1): 338–43.
5. Hesketh, P. J. Potential role of the NK1 receptor antagonists in chemotherapy-induced nausea and vomiting. Support Care Cancer 2001; 9(5): 350–4.
6. Twycross, R. *Pain Relief in Advanced Cancer*. 1994, Churchill Livingstone: London.
7. Malik, I. A. et al. Clinical efficacy of lorazepam in prophylaxis of anticipatory, acute, and delayed nausea and vomiting induced by high doses of cisplatin. A prospective randomized trial. Am J Clin Oncol 1995; 18(2): 170–5.
8. Priestman, T. J. et al. Results of a randomized, double-blind comparative study of ondansetron and metoclopramide in the prevention of nausea and vomiting following high-dose upper abdominal irradiation. Clin Oncol (R Coll Radiol) 1990; 2(2): 71–5.
9. Priestman, T. J., J. T. Roberts, et al. A prospective randomized double-blind trial comparing ondansetron versus prochlorperazine for the prevention of nausea and vomiting in patients undergoing fractionated radiotherapy. Clin Oncol 1993; 5(6): 358–63.
10. Roberts, J.T. and T.J. Priestman. A review of ondansetron in the management of radiotherapy-induced emesis. Oncology 1993; 50(3): 173–9.
11. Diemunsch, P. and L. Grelot. Potential of substance P antagonists as antiemetics. Drugs 2000; 60(3): 533–46.
12. Peroutka, S. J. and S. H. Snyder. Antiemetics: Neurotransmitter receptor binding predicts therapeutic actions. Lancet 1982; 1(8273): 658–9.
13. Terndrup, T. E. et al. Comparison of intramuscular meperidine and promethazine with and without chlorpromazine: A randomized, prospective, double-blind trial. Ann Emerg Med 1993; 22(2): 206–11.
14. Ernst, A. A. et al. Prochlorperazine versus promethazine for uncomplicated nausea and vomiting in the emergency department: A randomized, double-blind clinical trial. Ann Emerg Med 2000; 36(2): 89–94.
15. Bruera, E. and et al. Chronic nausea in advanced cancer patients: A retrospective assessment of metoclopramide-based anti-emetic regimen. J Pain Symptom Manage 1996; 11: 147–53.
16. Loewen, P. S., C. A. Marra, et al. 5-HT3 receptor antagonists vs traditional agents for the prophylaxis of postoperative nausea and vomiting. Can J Anaesth 2000; 47(10): 1008–18.

17. Hoskin, P. Radiotherapy in symptom management. In: D. Doyle, G. Hanks, et al., eds. *The Oxford Textbook of Palliative Medicine*. 1998, Oxford University Press: New York, pp. 267–82.

18. Kast, R. E. Mirtazapine may be useful in treating nausea and insomnia of cancer chemotherapy. Support Care Cancer 2001; 9(6): 469–70.

19. Tramer, M. R. et al. Cannabinoids for control of chemotherapy induced nausea and vomiting: Quantitative systematic review. BMJ 2001; 323(7303): 16–21.

20. Hallenbeck, J. and D. E. Weissman. Fast Fact and Concept #5: Treatment of nausea and vomiting. End of Life Education Project. http://www.eperc.mcw.edu/, 2000.

21. Enck, R. *The Medical Care of Terminally Ill Patients*. 1994, Johns Hopkins University Press: Baltimore, pp. 28–32.

22. Mancini, I. and E. Bruera. Constipation in advanced cancer patients. Support Care Cancer 1998; 6(4): 356–64.

23. Bruera, E. et al. The assessment of constipation in terminal cancer patients admitted to a palliative care unit: A retrospective review. J Pain Symptom Manage 1994; 9(8): 515–9.

24. Hallenbeck, J. and D. E. Weissman. Fast Fact and Concept #15; Constipation. End of Life Education Project. http://www.eperc.mcw.edu/, 2000.

25. Fallon, M. and B. O'Neill. ABC of palliative care. Constipation and diarrhoea. BMJ 1997; 315(7118): 1293–6.

26. Ahmedzai, S. and D. Brooks. Transdermal fentanyl versus sustained-release oral morphine in cancer pain: Preference, efficacy, and quality of life. The TTS-Fetanyl Comparative Trial Group. J Pain Symptom Manage 1997; 13: 254–61.

27. Radbruch, L. et al. Constipation and the use of laxatives: A comparison between transdermal fentanyl and oral morphine. Palliat Med 2000; 14: 111–9.

28. Hunt, R. et al. A comparison of subcutaneous morphine and fentanyl in hospice cancer patients. J Pain Symptom Manag 1999; 18: 111–9.

29. Hurdon, V., R. Viola, et al. How useful is docusate in patients at risk for constipation? A systematic review of the evidence in the chronically ill. J Pain Symptom Manage 2000; 19(2): 130–6.

30. Ripamonti, C. et al. Clinical-practice recommendations for the management of bowel obstruction in patients with end-stage cancer. Support Care Cancer 2001; 9(4): 223–33.

31. Beattie, G., F. Leonard, et al. Bowel obstruction in ovarian carcinoma: A retrospective study and review of the literature. Palliat Med 1981; 3: 275–80.

32. Baines, M., D. Oliver, et al. Medical management of intestinal obstruction in patients with advanced malignant disease: A clinical and pathologic study. Lancet 1985; ii: 990–3.

33. Welch, J. *Bowel Obstruction*. 1990, WB Saunders: Philadelphia.

34. Hutchison, S., G. Beattie, et al. Increased serotonin excretion in patients with ovarian carcinoma of the ovary. Palliat Med 1995; 9: 67–8.

35. Cubeddu, L. Serotonin mechanisms in chemotherapy-induced emesis in cancer patients. Oncology 1996; 53(suppl 1): 18–25.

36. Isbister, W., P. Elder, et al. Non-operative management of malignant intestinal obstruction. Journal of the Royal College of Physicians of Edinburgh 1990; 35: 369–72.

37. Ventafridda, V. et al. The management of inoperable gastrointestinal obstruction in terminal cancer patients. Tumori 1990; 76: 389–93.

38. Aranha, G., F. Folk, et al. Surgical palliation of small bowel obstruction due to metastatic carcinoma. Am Surg 1981; 13: 44–9.

39. Krebs, H. and D. Goplerud. The role of intestinal intubation in obstruction of the small intestine due to carcinoma of the ovary. Surgery, Gynecology, and Obstetrics 1984; 158: 467–71.
40. Bizar, L. et al. Small bowel obstruction. Surgery 1981; 89: 407–13.
41. Osteen, R. et al. Malignant intestinal obstruction. Surgery 1980; 67: 611–5.
42. De Conno, F. et al. Continuous subcutaneous infusion of hyscine butylbromide reduces secretions in patients with gastrointestinal obstruction. J Pain Symptom Manage 1991; 6: 484–6.
43. Hardy, J. et al. Pitfalls in placebo-controlled trials in palliative care: Dexamethasone for the palliation of malignant bowel obstruction. Palliat Med 1998; 9: 67–8.
44. Tuna, J., D. Buchler, et al. The management of ovarian-cancer-caused bowel obstruction. Gynecol Oncol 1981; 12: 186–92.
45. Soetikno, R., D. Lichtenstein, et al. Palliation of malginant gastric outlet obstruction using an endoscopically placed wallstent. Gastrointest Endosc 1998; 12: 267–70.
46. Friedland, S., J. Hallenbeck, et al. Stenting the sigmoid colon in a terminally ill patient with prostate cancer. Journal of Palliative Medicine 2001; 4(2): 153–6.
47. Mangli, G., M. Franchi, et al. Octreotide in the management of bowel obstruction in terminal ovarian cancer. Gynecol Oncol 1996; 61: 345–8.
48. Khoo, D., E. Hall, et al. Palliation of malignant intestinal obstruction using octreotide. Eur J Cancer 1994; 30: 28–30.
49. Mercadante, S. et al. Comparison of octreotide and hyoscine butylbromide in controlling gastrointestinal symptoms due to malignant inoperable bowel obstruction. Support Care Cancer 2000; 8(3): 188–91.
50. Ripamonti, C. et al. Role of octreotide, scopolamine butylbromide, and hydration in symptom control of patients with inoperable bowel obstruction and nasogastric tubes: A prospective randomized trial. J Pain Symptom Manage 2000; 19(1): 23–289.
51. Fainsinger, R. et al. Symptom control in terminally ill patients with malignant bowel obstruction. J Pain Symptom Manage 1994; 9: 12–8.
52. Feinle, C. and N. Read. Ondansetron reduces nausea induced by gastroduodenal stimulation without changing gastric motility. Am J Physiol 1996; 271: 6591–7.
53. Ventafridda, V. et al. Mouth care. In: D. Doyle, G. Hanks, et al., eds. The Oxford Textbook of Palliative Medicine. 1998, Oxford University Press: New York, pp. 691–8.
54. Ng, K. and C. F. von Gunten. Symptoms and attitudes of 100 consecutive patients admitted to an acute hospice/palliative care unit. J Pain Symptom Manage 1998; 16(5): 307–16.
55. McCann, R. M., W. J. Hall, et al. Comfort care for terminally ill patients. The appropriate use of nutrition and hydration. JAMA 1994; 272(16): 1263–6.
56. Stern, L. Preliminary study of glycopyrrolate in the management of drooling. J Paediatr Child Health 1997; 33: 52–4.
57. Olsen, A. K. and P. Sjogren. Oral glycopyrrolate alleviates drooling in a patient with tongue cancer. J Pain Symptom Manage 1999; 18: 300–2.
58. Ripamonti, C. and E. Bruera. Dyspnea: Pathophysiology and assessment. J Pain Symptom Manage 1997; 13(4): 220–32.
59. Reuben, D. B. and V. Mor. Dyspnea in terminally ill cancer patients. Chest 1986; 89(2): 234–6.
60. Bruera, E. et al. The frequency and correlates of dyspnea in patients with advanced cancer. J Pain Symptom Manage 2000; 19(5): 357–62.
61. Skilbeck, J. Palliative care in chronic obstructive airways disease: A needs assessment. Palliat Med 1998; 12: 245–54.

62. Watanabe, S. The role of oxygen in cancer-related dyspnea. In: R. Portenoy and E. Bruera, eds. *Topics in Palliative Care.* 2000, Oxford University Press: New York, pp. 255–60.

63. Bruera, E. et al. Effects of oxygen on dyspnoea in hypoxaemic terminal-cancer patients. Lancet 1993; 342(8862): 13–4.

64. American Thoracic Society. Dyspnea. Mechanisms, assessment, and management: A consensus statement. American Thoracic Society. Am J Respir Crit Care Med 1999; 159(1): 321–40.

65. Cristiano, L. M. and R. M. Schwartzstein. Effect of chest wall vibration on dyspnea during hypercapnia and exercise in chronic obstructive pulmonary disease. Am J Respir Crit Care Med 1997; 155(5): 1552–9.

66. Edo, H. et al. Effects of chest wall vibration on breathlessness during hypercapnic ventilatory response. J Appl Physiol 1998; 84(5): 1487–91.

67. Nakayama, H. et al. In-phase chest wall vibration decreases dyspnea during arm elevation in chronic obstructive pulmonary disease patients. Intern Med 1998; 37(10): 831–5.

68. Bruera, E. et al. Effects of morphine on the dyspnea of terminal cancer patients. J Pain Symptom Manage 1990; 5(6): 341–4.

69. Mazzocato, C., T. Buclin, et al. The effects of morphine on dyspnea and ventilatory function in elderly patients with advanced cancer: A randomized double-blind controlled trial. Ann Oncol 1999; 10(12): 1511–4.

70. Zeppetella, G. Nebulized morphine in the palliation of dyspnoea. Palliat Med 1997; 11: 267–73.

71. Chandler, S. Nebulized opioids to treat dyspnea. American Journal of Hospice & Palliative Care 1999; 16(1): 418–22.

72. Stark, R. D. et al. Effects of small-particle aerosols of local anaesthetic on dyspnoea in patients with respiratory disease. Clin Sci (Colch) 1985; 69(1): 29–36.

73. Libby, D., W. Briscoe, et al. Relief of hypoxia-related bronchoconstriction by breathing 30 percent oxygen. American Review of Respiratory Disease 1981; 123: 171–5.

74. Liss, H. and B. Grant. The effect of nasal flow on breathlessness in patients with chronic obstructive pulmonary disease. American Review of Respiratory Disease 1988; 137: 1285–8.

75. Brennan, M. F. Uncomplicated starvation versus cancer cachexia. Cancer Res 1977; 37(7 pt 2): 2359–64.

76. Dulloo, A. G., J. Jacquet, et al. Poststarvation hyperphagia and body fat overshooting in humans: A role for feedback signals from lean and fat tissues. Am J Clin Nutr 1997; 65(3): 717–23.

77. Alexander, H. Prevalence and pathophysiology of cancer cachexia. In: R. K. Portenoy and E. Bruera, eds. *Topics in Palliative Care.* 1998, Oxford University Press: New York, pp. 91–129.

78. Inui, A. Cancer anorexia-cachexia syndrome: Are neuropeptides the key? Cancer Res 1999; 59(18): 4493–501.

79. Dunlop, R. J. and C. W. Campbell. Cytokines and advanced cancer. J Pain Symptom Manage 2000; 20(3): 214–32.

80. Freeman, L. M. and R. Roubenoff. The nutrition implications of cardiac cachexia. Nutr Rev 1994; 52(10): 340–7.

81. Nemechek, P. M., B. Polsky, et al. Treatment guidelines for HIV-associated wasting. Mayo Clin Proc 2000; 75(4): 386–94.

82. Neuenschwander, H. and E. Bruera. Pathophysiology of cancer asthenia. In: R. K. Portenoy and E. Bruera, eds. *Topics in Palliative Care*. 1998, Oxford University Press: New York, pp. 171–81.
83. Cleary, J. F. The reversible causes of asthenia in cancer patients. In: R. K. Portenoy and E. Bruera, eds. *Topics in Palliative Care*. 1998, Oxford University Press: New York, pp. 183–202.
84. Vigano, A., S. Watanabe, et al. Anorexia and cachexia in advanced cancer patients. Cancer Surv 1994; 21: 99–115.
85. De Conno, F. et al. Megestrol acetate for anorexia in patients with far-advanced cancer: A double-blind controlled clinical trial. Eur J Cancer 1998; 34(11): 1705–9.
86. Yanagawa, H. et al. Palliative steroid therapy and serum interleukin-6 levels in a patient with lung cancer. J Pain Symptom Manage 1996; 12(3): 195–8.
87. Beal, J., R. Olson, et al. Dronabinol as treatment for anorexia associated with weight loss in patients with AIDS. J Pain Symptom Manage 1995; 10: 89.
88. Gleeson, C. Blood transfusion and its benefits in palliative care. Palliat Med 1995; 9(4): 307–13.

6

Special Therapeutic Issues: Hydration, Nutrition, and Antibiotics in End-of-Life Care

I have no pain, dear mother, now;
But oh! I am so dry:
Just moisten poor Jim's lips once more;
And, mother, do not cry!
                 Edward Farmer, 1809–76, *The Collier's Dying Child*

As in the case of Mr. A in the previous chapter, palliative care clinicians are frequently asked what they will or will not provide in terms of specific therapies. "Does your hospice allow IVs?" "You can't let Mom starve to death!" "He has pneumonia. You're giving him antibiotics, aren't you?" Chapter 8 on communication addresses how to respond to such inquiries in terms of communication skills. Here, I focus on the specific issues of hydration, nutrition, and antibiotics, issues that commonly arise at the end of life.

Hydration and Nutrition

The discussion of cachexia, anorexia, and asthenia in chapter 5 leads naturally to a broader discussion of the role of hydration and nutrition. Eating and drinking are the means to two overt goals: sustaining life through the provision of calories, nutrients, and water and the alleviation of suffering associated with hunger, thirst, and decreased functional status. Both eating and drinking also represent basic pleasures in life. Beyond this, eating and drinking are also social activities that offer opportunities for nurturing and for being nurtured. In everyday life we are largely unaware that separate goals exist; eating and drinking are simply good things to do. In palliative care distinctions between life-prolonging and life-enhancing goals are often required. Confusion about goals in this area causes a great deal of distress in palliative and end-of-life care.[1]

If the goals of care are directed solely to the provision of comfort (and enhancement of associated pleasures) and not life-prolongation, then a life-prolonging goal is no longer relevant. In such cases decisions regarding all forms of feeding should be assessed relative to the goals of alleviating suffering and enhancing quality of life. Natural but assisted feeding, such as spoon-feeding, may alleviate hunger or thirst and usually provides simple pleasure. As such, it may be welcomed. However, force-feeding, especially of patients who have lost their appetites and thirst, may, in fact, cause distress, usually at the hands of well-intentioned family members or caregivers who feel compelled to get some arbitrary amount of food into a patient. This compulsion usually arises from a lack of clarity in goals and from values that equate volume of intake with nurturing and quality of care.

Looking more closely at the issue of artificial hydration, like any therapy, it has potential benefits and burdens.[2–5] Most hospice practitioners believe that the burdens of artificial hydration at the very end of life outweigh the potential benefits. Dry mouth, as previously discussed, is a common problem, and true thirst may also be present, although studies suggest that thirst is less prevalent and troublesome than is dry mouth at the end of life and tends to fade near death.[6,7] However, there is little, if any, correlation between hydration status and both thirst and dry mouth at the end of life. For example, Ellershaw found in a prospective study no difference in the incidence of dry mouth or thirst between patients with normal hydration statuses as measured by serum osmolality and dehydrated patients.[8] Musgrave found no evidence of relief of dry mouth or thirst, if present, in patients in advanced stages of dying who were treated with intravenous therapy.[9] Ripamonti and colleagues, in a study that compared treatments of malignant bowel obstruction, found no statistical difference in daily thirst or dry mouth scores for patients who were receiving IV hydration (>2000 cc/d) compared to those not parenterally hydrated (<500 cc/d). (Interestingly, in this study hydrated patients experienced less nausea than did nonhydrated patients.)[10]

Many hospice workers believe hydration may worsen retained respiratory secretions at the very end of life. However, the effect of hydration on respiratory secretions at the end of life is unclear. Ellershaw found no correlation between hydration status and secretions in her study. None of the patients in that study were artificially hydrated.

It is clear that in some circumstances hydration can alleviate symptoms of delirium in dying patients.[11-14] However, it may be technically difficult to maintain IV or SC hydration in patients who have poor access or are agitated. Fussing over IVs or, worse, restraining patients to enable IV hydration can contribute significantly to suffering for patients and families. Although decisions must be individualized, in my experience most patients do quite well without hydration in advanced stages of dying.

My impression is that most hospice workers, having treated many patients with and without hydration at the end of life, would generally prefer not to receive hydration when their turns come. One study supports this view. Andrews and Levine surveyed 96 hospice nurses about their experiences and opinions on this matter. "Overall, the study showed that hospice nurses who were experienced in the matter of terminal dehydration viewed it as beneficial in the terminal stages of life."[15] That is, surveyed nurses favored not using artifical hydration.

In chapter 5 the limited effectiveness of artificial feeding was discussed relative to cachexia, anorexia, and asthenia. I now consider in more detail tube feeding as a means of providing hydration and nutrition. The following "Fast Fact" on tube feeding was generated to provide clinicians with some basic guidelines for their discussions and decision making with patients and families.[16] It is remarkable how often clinicians suggest tube feeding or place tubes with no data to support the purported goals of therapy.

Tube Feed or Not Tube Feed? [adapted from 16]

Tube feeding is frequently used in chronically ill and dying patients. The evidence base for much of this use is weak at best. In the list below some of what is known (and not known) is summarized about tube feeding for specific indications.

For prevention of aspiration pneumonia

- Reduction in the chance of pneumonia has been suggested for nonbedridden post-stroke patients in one prospective, nonrandomized study. For bedridden post-stroke patients, no reduction was observed.[17] Three retrospective cohort studies that compared patients with and without tube feeding demonstrated no advantage to tube feeding for this purpose.
- Swallowing studies, such as videofluoroscopy, lack both sensitivity and specificity in predicting who will develop aspiration pneumonia. Croghan's study of 22 patients who underwent videofluoroscopy demonstrated a sensitivity of 65% and specificity of 67% in predicting who would develop aspiration pneumonia within one year.[18] In this study no reduction in the incidence of pneumonia was demonstrated in those who were tube fed.
- Swallowing studies may be helpful in providing guidance regarding swallowing techniques for populations amenable to instruction.

- Numerous observational studies have shown a high incidence of aspiration pneumonia in those who have been tube fed.

For life prolongation via caloric support

- Data is strongest for patients with reversible illnesses who are in a catabolic state (such as acute sepsis).
- Data is weakest in advanced cancer. No improvement in survival has been found (with the few exceptions noted below).
- Nonrandomized retrospective and prospective studies have found no survival advantage in patients with advanced dementia.
- Tube feeding may be life-prolonging in select circumstances in chronic illness: patients with proximal GI obstruction due to cancer and a high functional status, patients receiving chemotherapy/XRT involving the proximal GI tract, certain patients with AIDS, and those with amyotrophic lateral sclerosis.

For enhancing quality of life

- When true hunger and thirst exist, quality of life may be enhanced (such as in very proximal GI obstruction).
- Most actively dying patients do *not* experience hunger or thirst (although dry mouth is a common problem).
- Dry mouth is *not* improved by tube feeding (or IV hydration).
- A recent literature review using *palliative care* and *enteral nutrition* as search terms found no studies that demonstrate improved quality of life through tube feeding. (Limited to a few observational studies.)
- Tube feeding may adversely affect quality of life if patients are denied the pleasure of eating.

It is important to understand that tube feeding should always be considered relative to patient goals. Physicians should be prepared to discuss tube feeding as an option bearing in mind what evidence (or lack thereof) exists that tube feeding will help reach such goals.[15,18-20]

Tube feeding can be extremely helpful for patients with acute medical problems and for certain patients with chronic illnesses such as amyotrophic lateral sclerosis who want and need nutritional support. However, the benefit of tube feeding in most advanced and terminal illnesses is less clear. A large observational study of more than 7000 patients who received PEG (percutaneous endoscopic gastrostomy) tubes found that the three top reasons for PEG tube placement were organic neurologic disorders such as dementia (29%), stroke (19%), and head and neck cancer (16%). Of these, 24% of patients died during the hospitalization in which a PEG tube was placed, and median survival was 7.5 months.[21] Meier and colleagues followed 99 patients with advanced dementia who were hospitalized. A new tube for feeding was given to 50%. Only 37%

left without a tube (17% came and left with a tube). Median survival for all patients followed was 175 days, with no statistically significant difference in survival for patients who received tube feeding compared to those not tube fed ($p = .90$).[22] Thus, in patients with advanced dementia, who undergo PEG tube placement with remarkable frequency, there is no evidence for life prolongation.

What about quality of life? Few studies have been done. A small study of 150 patients chronically tube fed in a community cohort study found no evidence of improvement in functional status, nutritional status, or quality of life when followed prospectively. As in the other studies cited above, mortality was approximately 50% at one year.[23]

The list above briefly discusses the use of tube feeding for the prevention of aspiration pneumonia and points out that evidence to support this common practice is very limited. Although some benefit may exist for mild to moderate post-stroke patients, there is no evidence of benefit in patients with very advanced illness due to strokes who are bedridden.

Often, patients thought to be at risk for aspiration undergo videofluoroscopy to look for evidence of food "going down the wrong way." Based on this, it has become common practice to recommend tube feeding for those patients who demonstrate aspiration. It seems to make sense. Food going down the wrong way is a bad thing. It would seem that if we just bypass this problem, everything will be alright. This seems to be the story upon which clinicians justify this very common chain of events—except that there is no evidence that this helps most patients. It is worth noting that videofluoroscopy was never developed as a predictive test for aspiration pneumonia; it was developed to help speech therapists understand the physiology of swallowing disorders for the purpose of assisting therapists in training patients in new ways of swallowing. Apparently, it works well for this purpose. Clinicians who perform videofluoroscopy found patients with evidence of food "going down the wrong way" and felt they had to do something.

How can we make sense of the findings to date (admittedly based on limited studies) that NG and PEG tubes do *not* decrease the incidence of aspiration pneumonia in most cases? While more studies would be helpful, perhaps we should consider some alternative stories. Why might tube feeding *not* decrease the risk of pneumonia and why might it *not* prolong survival? First, by bypassing eating we have overridden a whole host of feedback mechanisms that inform people whether their stomachs are empty or full. *Override* risks *overflow* (regurgitation with aspiration and diarrhea). Second, the functioning of the upper intestinal tract appears to be profoundly affected. The physical presence of the tube increases the risk of reflux by inhibiting normal motility, which contributes to the problem of overflow.[24] Finally, we might challenge the assumption that aspiration pneumonia is tightly linked to aspiration of food, as demonstrated on videofluoroscopy. Although, arguably, bypassing the system may decrease the probability of *food* aspiration, patients may still aspirate saliva, which contains large numbers of bacteria. This cannot be prevented. My sense is that for most patients aspiration pneumonia is not so much a disease to be prevented as it is a sign of often unrecognized global physiologic decline. The immune system is often compromised for reasons other than malnutrition, and this makes the patient more susceptible to infections. Because of general weakness and inhibition of the cough reflex, patients often cannot clear their airways of secretions, and this increases the probability of pneumonia. None of these problems are correctable by tube placement.

Why, then, despite the lack of evidence in most cases for efficacy relative to the goals of life prolongation and improved quality of life, has tube feeding persisted in its popularity? A basic reason is that clinicians and families have not seriously questioned the common story line that assumes that not eating and drinking is simply a mechanical problem that can be solved by bypassing the normal intake mechanism. Callahan examined the decision-making processes that resulted in PEG tube placement in 100 patients using questionnaires and semistructured interviews. Tube placement usually occurred in the midst of acute decompensations that elicited much distress on the part of clinicians, patients, and families. The major finding of this study was that "Patients, caregivers, and physicians are often compelled to make decisions about long-term enteral feeding under tragic circumstances and with incomplete information. Decision-makers typically do not perceive any acceptable alternatives." Decisions for tube feeding were usually "nondecisions" that proceeded along set story lines that went unquestioned. "Physicians have clear patterns of triage for percutaneous endoscopic gastrostomy, but the assumptions underlying these patterns are not well supported by the medical literature."[25] The underlying issue seems less medical than cultural and psychological.

Often, I find myself in the position of recommending against therapies such as tube feeding when I believe they will not be beneficial to the patient. To the best of my ability, I try to explain what is known and not known about the potential benefits and burdens of tube feeding. However, given that this is a culturally and psychologically loaded issue, families very often have trouble accepting my story, which seems so at odds with their own story lines. In listening to their stories about why they think artificial nutrition is needed, I am struck by how much is *assumed* (for example, that bypassing the system will automatically fix the problem or that not feeding artificially is the equivalent of starvation) and by how little insight people often have into the psychological processes that frequently underlie their requests. (The same can be said for clinicians.) As I will discuss further in Chapter 8 on communication, if my explanation, my story, of why I believe artificial hydration or nutrition would not be beneficial is understood simply as an invalidation their stories, it will, quite reasonably, be rejected. The trick, which is far easier said than done, seems to be to validate those elements in the family (or clinician) story line that make sense, at least in terms of intent, and try to reframe, or at least suggest alternative interpretations (such as understanding that not feeding does not equal starvation), in terms of their story line. In Table 6.1, in abbreviated fashion, I outline how this might be done for a request for artificial nutrition when I believe it would not be helpful.

Antibiotics

The use of antibiotics for bacterial infections is considered routine by many. Clinicians and lay people often view the withholding of antibiotics in the presence of bacterial infection as de facto neglect. On the other hand, some clinicians who refer patients to palliative care units or hospices still sometimes ask if their patients can receive antibiotics under the assumption that antibiotics are prohibited. This is not (or should not) be true. As for any other therapy, the real issue is the *intent* in giving antibiotics and whether antibiotics will be helpful in reaching certain goals.

Antibiotics may affect both the quality and quantity of life in complex ways.[26] To the extent that antibiotics can help clear an infection that results in pneumonia even transiently, quality of life may be enhanced relative to that particular episode of pneumonia. Dyspnea, cough, fever, and delirium may all improve if the patient recovers. The use of antibiotics on the other hand, may adversely affect quality of life in that suppressing an existing infection without cure sometimes merely prolongs an acute, uncomfortable dying process from a day or two to several days. Even if a terminal patient briefly recovers, recurrent infection may result. In summing up the suffering inherent in (potentially) several such episodes before eventual death, the net quality of life may be worse with treatment than without. Antibiotics may have significant side effects, such as *Clostridium difficile* diarrhea caused by bacterial overgrowth as the normal gut flora is killed. Such side effects have a directly adverse effect on quality of life.

Antibiotics may or may not prolong life. It is almost a truism to point out that the closer a patient is to death, the less effect antibiotics will have on prolonging life. This has been best demonstrated for patients with Alzheimer's dementia.[27] Volicer showed no significant difference in mortality of advanced Alzheimer patients treated for febrile episodes with or without antibiotics. For patients more mildly demented, there was a survival advantage to antibiotics. Studies are generally lacking for other terminal illnesses. However, the same principle seems to apply: the closer to death a patient is, the less difference antibiotics will make in prolonging life.

Whether life prolongation per se is seen as a benefit or burden will vary with the individual. Some patients will see any prolongation as a distinct burden. Even transient life prolongation, if possible, may be meaningful for others.

TABLE 6.1. Reframing Requests for Artificial Nutrition

FAMILY UNDERSTANDING	RESPONSE	COMMENT
He is dying because he is not able to eat or drink.	A) I understand how worrisome that must be.	A) Empathetic validation of concern.
	B) Of course, it must seem that getting food and water into him would be important.	B) Validation that their explanation, if true, would suggest the appropriateness of artificial nutrition.
	C) We have noticed that he only wants small amounts of food and water.	C) Drawing attention to information available to suggest an alternative explanation.
	D) People with this illness who are dying tend not to be hungry or thirsty.	D) Sharing alternative explanation that validates linkage between nutrition and dying, but in a different way, thereby reframing the issue.
We can't let him starve to death (die of thirst), which can be prevented by artificial feeding.	A) You are right, if he were starving or thirsty and we could prolong his life through such feeding, that would make sense.	A) Validation of internal consistency of their story.
	B) While it may seem like starvation, what is going on is somewhat different. . . .	B) Suggest possible alternative interpretation.
	C) It would be great if tube feeding worked that way. However, in other patients with this illness we have found that tube feeding neither prolongs life nor makes people feel better.	C) Share more information that suggests that tube feeding will not accomplish their goals, which are reasonable in and of themselves.
So we're just going to do nothing	A) Not at all! This is a time to pay special attention. . . .	A) Acknowledge "need to nurture" and reframe current situation in terms of this.
	B) He may not be able to eat or drink much, but is there some special food he really liked?	B) Involve family (facilitating nurturing) concretely in a new way—feeding for pleasure vs. calories
	C) At this stage dry mouth is a big problem. You could really help us care for him by giving . . . (ice chips, swabs, lemon drops, etc.).	C) Identify how family can be of help in paying special attention, thereby forming an alliance.

There are a number of situations in which antibiotics are clearly palliative. Pains of sinusitis, dental abscess, cellulitis, and parotitis, for example, are best treated with antibiotics, not morphine. These infections rarely cause death. The relative benefit or burden of life prolongation is not an issue.

At times, antibiotic therapy will appear to the clinician to be medically futile. That is, relative to certain goals (whether symptom relief or life prolongation), antibiotics will be judged to be ineffective. Once possible benefits (or lack thereof) and burdens have been raised, some will remain adamant in their demands that antibiotics be given. Patients and families may get stuck on a particular therapy such as antibiotics and be unable to get beyond what is often medically a rather trivial issue. In many such cases the relative harm of antibiotic administration to the dying patient is often minimal, as is the probability of medical response. In such cases the clinician may consider giving antibiotics (or similar therapies) in recognition that such requests arise out of psychological and cultural needs. The intent in such an approach is to remove the obstructing issue in the hope that the patient and family can move on to the more important work of coping with the impending loss of the patient. Physicians may be fearful that one request will lead only to increasingly unreasonable requests. Although this can happen, in my experience it is more likely that demonstrating flexibility will be appreciated and will enhance the relationship. Beneath most requests for antibiotics is a simple desire for provision of the best possible care and a hope that we not abandon the patient. If we can convince patients and families of this, we will establish an enduring relationship beneficial to all.

References

1. Huang, Z. B. and J. C. Ahronheim. Nutrition and hydration in terminally ill patients: An update. Clin Geriatr Med 2000; 16(2): 313–25.
2. Printz. Terminal dehydration, a compassionate treatment. Arch Intern Med 1992; 152: 697–700.
3. McCann, R. and W. Hall. Comfort care for terminally ill patients. JAMA 1994; 272: 1263–6.
4. Dunphy, K. Rehydration in palliative and terminal care: If not–why not? Palliative Medicine 1995; 9: 221–8.
5. Ahronheim, J. Nutrition and hydration in the terminal patient. Clin Geriatr Med 1996; 12: 379–91.
6. Burge, F. I. Dehydration symptoms of palliative care cancer patients. J Pain Symptom Manage 1993; 8(7): 454–64.
7. Conill, C., et al. Symptom prevalence in the last week of life. J Pain Symptom Manage, 1997; 14(6): 328–31.
8. Ellershaw, J., J. Sutcliff, et al. Dehydration and the dying patient. J Pain Symptom Manage 1995; 10: 192–7.
9. Musgrave, C. F., N. Bartal, et al. The sensation of thirst in dying patients receiving i.v. hydration. J Palliat Care 1995; 11(4): 17–21.

10. Ripamonti, C. et al. Role of octreotide, scopolamine butylbromide, and hydration in symptom control of patients with inoperable bowel obstruction and nasogastric tubes: A prospective randomized trial. J Pain Symptom Manage 2000; 19(1): 23–289.

11. Fainsinger, R. and E. Bruera. When to treat dehydration in a terminally ill patient. Support Care Cancer 1997; 5: 205–11.

12. Fainsinger, R. L. Treatment of delirium at the end of life: Medical and ethical issues. In: R.K. Portenoy and E. Bruera, eds. Topics in Palliative Care. 1998, Oxford University Press: New York, pp. 261–77.

13. Lawlor, P. G., R. L. Fainsinger, et al. Delirium at the end of life: Critical issues in clinical practice and research. JAMA 2000; 284(19): 2427–9.

14. Lawlor, P. and B. Gagnon. Occurrence, causes, and outcomes of delirium in patients with advanced cancer: A prospective study. Arch Intern Med 2000; 160: 786–94.

15. Andrews, M. and A. Levine. Dehydration in the terminal patient: Perception of hospice nurses. American Journal of Hospice Care 1989; 6: 31–4.

16. Hallenbeck, J. and D. E. Weissman. Fast Fact and Concept #10: Tube feed or not tube feed. End of Life Education Project. http://www.eperc.mcw.edu/, 2000.

17. Nakajoh, K. et al. Relation between incidence of pneumonia and protective reflexes in post- stroke patients with oral or tube feeding. J Intern Med 2000; 247(1): 39–42.

18. Croghan, J. et al. Pilot study of 12-month outcomes of nursing home patients with aspiration on videofluroscopy. Dysphagia 1994; 9: 141–6.

19. Finucane, T., C. Christmas, et al. Tube feeding in patients with advanced dementia. JAMA 1999; 282: 1365–9.

20. Finucane, T. and J. Bynum. Use of tube feeding to prevent aspiration pneumonia. Lancet 1996; 348: 1421–4.

21. Rabeneck, L., N. P. Wray, et al. Long-term outcomes of patients receiving percutaneous endoscopic gastrostomy tubes. J Gen Intern Med 1996; 11(5): 287–93.

22. Meier, D. E. et al. High short-term mortality in hospitalized patients with advanced dementia: Lack of benefit of tube feeding. Arch Intern Med 2001; 161(4): 594–9.

23. Callahan, C. M. et al. Outcomes of percutaneous endoscopic gastrostomy among older adults in a community setting. J Am Geriatr Soc 2000; 48(9): 1048–54.

24. Esparza, J. et al. Equal aspiration rates in gastrically and transpylorically fed critically ill patients. Intensive Care Med 2001; 27(4): 660–4.

25. Callahan, C. M. et al. Decision-making for percutaneous endoscopic gastrostomy among older adults in a community setting. J Am Geriatr Soc 1999; 47(9): 1105–9.

26. Freer, J. and D. Bentley. The role of antibiotics in comfort care. In: E. Olson, E. Chichin, et al., eds. Controversies in Ethics in Long-Term Care. 1995, Springer: New York, pp. 91–107.

27. Volicer, L. et al. Hospice approach to the treatment of patients with advanced dementia of the Alzheimer type. JAMA 1986; 256: 2210–3.

7

Psychosocial and Spiritual Aspects of Care

There is a time of the night between midnight and dawn when
people despair.

Anatole Broyard, *Intoxicated by My Illness*

Imagine that you are dying. Magically, you are completely comfortable, at least
physically, yet this is not your fantasy death. This is *not* how you want to die.
Where are you? What is happening? Why, despite being physically comfortable,
is this a death to be feared?

This exercise is the mirror image of the fantasy death exercise introduced in
the Chapter 2. When I do this educational exercise with clinicians, a heavy silence usually falls upon the group. No nervous laughter or jokes intrude. A soft
voice says, "In an ICU, hooked up to tubes." "Alone," echoes another. "In a
nursing home, tied down in bed." "In diapers." "In a dark room. Nobody else is
there—no family, no friends."

Difficult as this exercise is, I hope that through it participants come to understand the importance of the *psyche* at the end of life; there is far more to palliative care than treating physical symptoms. Although physical symptoms can be
very troublesome for dying patients, we are reasonably good at making such
symptoms at least bearable. My impression is that far more suffering in patients
with advanced illness results from psychic than from physical distress. I find such

127

distress much more challenging to address. Speaking just for myself—of course I *want* to be comfortable physically, but what I *fear* in my death is isolation.

Our language fails us in trying to put into words the psychic distress to which we bear witness. Categories of psychic distress tend to be extrapolated from formal psychological diagnoses. We speak of depression, anxiety, and delirium, for example. Such categorizations can be helpful in suggesting certain therapeutic approaches and will be discussed in more detail. However, when discussing psychic distress in advanced illness in particular, I often get the uneasy feeling that our definitions and categories sometimes fall short, better serving *our* need to impose organization on the mysterious landscape of the mind than necessarily serving our ability to aid the dying and their families.

A particular conundrum is to determine what is *normal* and what is *pathologic*—what is a normal part of the dying process and what is illness. The situation is much clearer with physical symptoms. We work with the assumption that symptoms such as chronic pain, nausea, and dyspnea are *not* normal and should be eliminated if at all possible. It is much harder to say what is normal in encountering a person in tears. Is this a good cry, reflecting healthy grief and acceptance, or evidence of pathologic depression? Can grief be abnormal? I believe grief can be pathologic, but it is hard to say exactly where the line is that distinguishes the normal from the abnormal.

Beyond the normal–abnormal dichotomy, we tend to characterize episodes of distress as problems separate from the person. Depression, anxiety, and delirium, for example, are viewed as *things* that can be fixed or removed. Again, there is some usefulness to such classification. However, this approach may blind us to the fact that psychic distress is intimately intertwined with personhood. If we consider common fears associated with dying, we find themes that do not so easily fit into neat diagnostic boxes. What is it people fear in their dying? Being alone? Separation and isolation? Not being in control? Living or having lived a life without meaning? These and related questions arise from the person and defy disease-oriented classification.

In the fantasy death exercise above, people tend to talk easily about where they do not want to be when they die—the ICU, a nursing home, and similar places. It may be difficult to acknowledge that these places (at least at a fantasy level) are also projections of *internal* fears that reflect threats to self as much as undesirable external circumstances. Other than the wrenching agony of acute loss, the greatest suffering I have witnessed in dying people and their families relates to perceived loss of control and isolation. This is admittedly a gross generalization and probably reflects our American culture's obsession with being in control. I cannot say how unique this is to our corner of the world. I suspect that at some basic level, not being able to live as one would like is a fairly universal form of suffering. To the extent this is true, why do we see so little discussion of this in palliative care education? I have reviewed many curricula for end-of-life care. Almost all contain something on depression and delirium but very little on the subjects of control and isolation per se. Why? My guess is that it has something to do with the fact that we do not categorize isolation or a "need to be in control" as illnesses. If we recognize suffering that appears to result from frustration in not being in control, we tend to see the issue as one of unavoidable external circumstances interacting with a relatively fixed personality. To the extent that we can modify the environment or the person's ability to interact with the environment, control can be enhanced and distress relieved. This can, in fact, be a very useful approach to such distress, but it is inherently limited by our ability to alter the environment or the person's ability to interact with the environment.

At deeper levels it may be difficult for palliative care clinicians to acknowledge that certain forms of psychic distress and suffering are beyond our control as clinicians. We like to be able to be fix things. We can treat certain manifestations of suffering such as anxiety and depression with a pill, but we may not get to the heart of the matter, because that "heart" is part of the *person*. This does not mean that we do nothing and can be of no assistance. However, it is a mistake to see such suffering as something separate from the person that is our job to fix or cure. To the extent we can support people in dealing with their suffering, relief can be found. Some forms of healing for suffering are to be found only within the person.

In keeping with the story theme of this book, how can we understand such distress? People have an understanding of how they got where they are at any given time. This understanding is part of their story, which projects into the future along a particular story line in a semicoherent manner. Thus, a person who sees his or her role in the story as a "fighter" will project this role into the future, even when there is a significant "turn in the plot," as often happens with illness.[1] This is one way of coping with an unexpected turn of events—we fall back on our strengths. However, at times people encounter plot changes that are so extreme that they appear to negate the very premises upon which their life stories have been built. The rugged individualist who prided himself on being able to handle any problem finds himself completely unprepared for life following a stroke. A mother of great religious faith looses a child, a loss that seems completely unfair and contrary to her belief in a just God. The daughter who swore she would never put her father in a nursing home finds she has no other recourse. In the aftermath she experiences crushing guilt.

The story lines of the rugged individualist, the person of faith, and the loyal daughter all contain admirable qualities and probably served these individuals well, but they may be inadequate, in and of themselves, to enable the protagonists to respond positively to new and unanticipated challenges that may arise associated with serious illness and death. People in such circumstances face crises in their story lines.

What are our roles as clinicians in all this? The truth is, we will find many people who will suffer mightily despite our best efforts. If we judge ourselves based on whether we can eliminate all suffering, we make the same mistake clinicians make when they judge death to be a failure because they could not cure everything. To the extent that a patient's or family member's distress arises from his or her story line, we must first approach this distress with respect. To negate the story line is tantamount to negating the person. If somebody really wants to die "with his boots on" or "rage, rage, against the dying of the light," I guess that is OK. At least he got to do it "his way" as Frank Sinatra crooned. I may be saddened by what I see, even think some of it foolish. However, I also feel I must struggle to respect that these are *their* stories, not mine. At times we will have special opportunities to suggest different approaches that may result in less distress and yet be acceptable within that person's story line. Rugged individualism may be reinterpreted as a strong spirit overcoming great obstacles such as increasing dependence. The care received in dependence may come to be understood as "getting one's due" after a life well-lived rather than as an assault on dignity.

Although I am warning against a rigid categorization of psychic distress, categories do help us understand certain patterns of distress and suggest certain approaches to the relief of suffering. I now consider some of these traditional categories.

Depression

"She's dying. Who wouldn't be depressed?" Reactions such as this are common when depression is encountered in the terminally ill. Depression at the end of life is estimated to occur in between 25% to 75% of cases; not rare, but also not inevitable. Even so, it is underrecognized by clinicians who may think that depression is part of normal dying. It is important to diagnose depression when it exists because depression is usually treatable.[2]

Diagnosing depression in dying patients can be tricky. The signs and symptoms clinicians have learned to associate with depression are unreliable in the dying. Vegetative signs and symptoms, such as anorexia, anhedonia, social withdrawal, and weight loss, may represent depression but may also occur in patients with pain, in grieving patients, and even in the "normally dying." Frequently, depression, grief, pain, and "normal dying" overlap.[3] The problem facing the clinician is not so much differential diagnosis in the traditional sense as it is to understand the relative contribution of various factors, such as depression, grief, and pain, to the patient's distress.

Standard instruments used to diagnose depression, such as the Geriatric Depression Scale (GDS), may be unreliable in dying patients because these instruments have not been rigorously tested in this population. The GDS was developed for geriatric patients in recognition of the fact that the functional measures of standard scales were found to be unhelpful in geriatric patients, who frequently have functional impairments that result from medical illness.[4] However, the GDS was not developed with dying in mind. GDS items such as, "I have crying spells" or "I feel hopeful about the future" may be interpreted very differently by dying patients. Some dying patients who score as depressed on the GDS may not actually be depressed. Tears may represent normal, healthy grief as well as depression. Concern about the future is fairly common among dying patients. We will one day have a valid instrument for discerning depression in dying patients. Until then, some suggested questions for evaluating depression at the end of life are:

- "Do you find yourself depressed most of the time?" This question attempts to address the fact that depression, unlike grief, tends to persist over time.
- "Compared to other people in similar situations, do you feel that you are depressed?" This question introduces a normative comparison to other seriously ill patients. This may help improve accuracy.
- "Inside yourself, how do you feel about yourself?" This question attempts to reveal poor self-esteem and associated worthlessness that are believed to be fairly reliable indicators of depression at the end of life.

My impression is that if patients say they are depressed in response to any of these or similar questions, they probably are depressed, as Chochinov and colleagues found in one study.[5] That is, these questions probably have good specificity, although they may lack sensitivity. I have certainly encountered a number of patients who seem unable to identify depression in themselves: "I don't know doctor, I just feel terrible all over . . ." My guess is that for these patients, a more structured instrument may be helpful in identifying clinical depression.

I will not try to pretend that I understand *why* people become depressed at the end of life or to what extent depression represents a biochemical imbalance. Certain risk factors for depression are known: a prior history of depression, poorly controlled pain, multiple losses, and certain disease processes such as hypothyroidism, pancreatic cancer, and stroke, among others.[6] Even though a prior history of depression is a rather obvious risk factor for depression, it is unclear to me that this necessarily means that the *severity* of depression will be worse for such patients at the end of life. I have met a number of patients with prior histories of depression who have learned to monitor their symptoms and to cope with depression when it occurs. Such patients may do quite well. In contrast, patients with no prior history of depression may be overwhelmed by new-onset depression, lack the coping skills for it, and experience more severe symptomatology. This would be an interesting research topic.

Whatever the cause, it is important not to view depression at the end of life simply as an unfortunate and random event, external to the person, to be solved simply with medication. Depression is usually heavily invested with meaning. In dying, unresolved issues commonly resurface. Coping strategies that might have served well in the past may not serve so well when confronted with dying. Fear may pervade depression. Often such fears go unspoken. "I may have accepted that I'm dying, but I'm terrified of what will happen. Nobody has spoken to me about that. . . ." The dying may also have fears for loved ones who will be left behind. "I just don't know how she is going to get by without me. . . ." Identifying these concerns and addressing them (in addition to treating other unrelieved symptoms such as pain) can go far in resolving depression.

Pharmacologic Treatment of Depression

For several reasons, the pharmacologic treatment of depression in dying patients is particularly challenging:[7]

- Patients may be unable to swallow or retain medications due to dysphagia, nausea, and emesis.
- Patients may have less ability to cope with adverse side effects of medications due to their illness. Dry mouth, for example, is common in dying patients and is exacerbated by antidepressants with anticholinergic properties.
- Treatment of depression in dying patients is often a race against time. At the time of evaluation patients may have a life expectancy of days to weeks. The latency period of antidepressants, the time it takes for them to "kick in," may consume a significant portion of the patient's remaining life.

Depressed patients often need multimodal therapy that combines psychosocial interventions with pharmacotherapy.

Pharmacotherapy

Drug therapy should be tailored to the individual patient's situation. Relevant questions to ask in comparing medications include:[8,9]

1. How long is the patient likely to live?
2. What side effects do you wish to avoid?
3. What side effects might enhance the patient's quality of life?

Psychostimulants. Psychostimulants such as methylphenidate and dextroamphetamine may be helpful when a rapid response (within 24 to 48 hours) is desired. They work best in patients with psychomotor retardation and should be avoided in agitated or confused patients. Positive side effects may include increased energy and appetite and counteraction of opioid-induced sedation. Psychostimulants may be continued indefinitely alone or with a selective serotonin reuptake inhibitor, and should be tapered off when they are being discontinued. Adverse effects include tremulousness, anxiety, and insomnia, although these are rarely seen with lower doses in most patients.[10]

Tricyclic antidepressants (TCAs). TCAs can serve a dual purpose as antidepressants and as analgesics in the treatment of neuropathic pain. Because of their anticholinergic properties they must be used with caution in the elderly. TCAs have a delayed onset of action for depression (two to four weeks) and have extensive drug–drug interactions. Of the TCAs, nortriptyline and desipramine have fewer anticholinergic effects than does amitriptyline, and renal clearance is less variable with age.[11] Notably, the antidepressant and analgesic effects of TCAs are not related their anticholinergic side effects. Therefore, unless anticholinergic side effects are explicitly desired (which is rare), TCAs with fewer anticholinergic side effects are generally preferred.

Selective serotonin reuptake inhibitors (SSRIs). The SSRIs have now become the first line of treatment for depression because of their safety profile, once-daily dosing schedule, and more rapid onset of action compared to TCAs (10 days to 2 weeks). In patients who are moderately to severely depressed, an SSRI may be given concomitantly with a psychostimulant, and the psychostimulant can be tapered off after one to two weeks if affect has improved.

Atypical antidepressants. A variety of "atypical" antidepressants are on the market. Here I discuss just one, trazodone. Its sedative properties are advantageous in treating depressed patients with insomnia. It is commonly used as a sleeping pill by geriatricians and appears to be especially useful in confused or demented patients with a tendency toward nocturnal confusion (sundowning). This drug is well tolerated by the elderly. Priapism is very rarely a concern in these patients.

Anxiety

Anxiety in dying patients tends to look very much like anxiety in patients who are not dying. Patients tend to be agitated. They may pace, call out, fidget, or moan. Anxiety is relatively easy to recognize. It is more difficult to understand *why* the patient is anxious. Anxiety can result from fears, grief reactions, or altered states of consciousness. It may be associated with physical symptoms, especially dyspnea and pain. Depression may also present with anxiety as a prominent feature.

Anxiety commonly arises in the dying. Although anxiety tends to respond to the usual anxiolytics, the clinician is cautioned not to jump to medications too quickly. Anxiety in most patients seems to be a transient state, and to reflect some deeper distress that we should try to identify and address. For most people dying is very scary. The images we have of dying, largely derived from movies and television, are ones of violence and pain. The fear of loss of self in dying is something people who know they are dying wrestle with, some more successfully than others. While there is no easy fix for such existential distress, many fears are very concrete and can be addressed, thereby relieving fear and associated anxiety. How will I die? Will it hurt? We can do much to reassure patients and families that most dying people who receive good palliative care die peacefully and that pain can be controlled. Identifying and addressing these fears, which are so scary to some that they have trouble verbalizing them, can go far toward relieving anxiety.

Anxiety related to grief may respond to grief facilitation (see section on grief below). Anxiety related to depression or physical symptoms often responds to treatment for depression or to relief of the physical symptom. Anxiety associated with altered states, such as sundowning in dementia, may improve if the sensorium is cleared using an agent such as haloperidol or by using reorienting activities such as pointing out clocks and familiar objects.

Pharmacotherapy for Anxiety

Benzodiazepines are the mainstay of pharmacotherapy for anxiety.[8] These medications can be very efficacious but should be used with caution, especially in the elderly when anxiety or agitation is thought to arise from dementia or delirium, because a "paradoxical response" may occur. Benzodiazepines can disinhibit patients, especially if they are prone to confusion. Benzodiazepines function rather like alcohol; one drink, and some people are swinging from the rafters, four drinks, and they are asleep. Lorazepam is most commonly used, as it is relatively short acting. If anxiety is responsive to benzodiazepines and is persistent throughout the day, a longer-acting agent, such as diazepam, may be chosen, much as we use long-acting opioids for basal pain.

Three other agents bear mentioning. Buspirone is a nonbenzodiazepine anxiolytic agent that can be helpful in certain cases. Its greatest disadvantage is its delayed onset of action, approximately two weeks. It may be considered for people with persistent anxiety who have a life expectancy of at least several weeks. Gabapentin is an anticonvulsant commonly used in the treatment of neuropathic pain. It also has anxiolytic properties and may be a useful agent for patients with anxiety who also have seizures or neuropathic pain.[12,13] Certain SSRI antidepressants such as paroxetine and mirtazapine have anxiolytic effects and may be of particular help in panic disorders.[14,15] Anxiety may also exist as a part of a continuum with terminal distress or delirium. The goal of standard anxiolytic therapy is to relieve anxiety without undue sedation. Unfortunately, in patients close to death, sometimes we have little choice but to advance to frank sedation if anxiety or agitation is unresponsive to standard anxiolytic doses. (See the discussion of treatment options in the section on altered states below.)

Grief

The longer I work in palliative care, the more I appreciate grief.[16] We tend to have a narrow concept of grief: someone dies, someone grieves. In fact, grief as a process seems central to human adaptation to the inevitability of change. Grief is usually the major issue for those who have lost a loved one. This is the grief of *bereavement*, yet we all grieve when we loose something or someone to whom we are attached. In seeing my grey and disappearing hair, I grieve my youth. I grieve the loss of a great nurse on our unit who just moved on to a new job. Even if they never treat a dying patient, clinicians come up against grief every day, whether they recognize it or not.

Several years ago, after lifting a heavy patient during an emergency, I noticed that one of my calves seemed a bit swollen and tender. I had also recently taken a long car trip. I imagined the worst: a deep vein thrombosis (DVT). I went to the ER to get an ultrasound of my leg. Over the next few hours I experienced an acute grief reaction. Anticipating a DVT, I looked into a future ruled by anticoagulants. How my life would change! I would have to be careful about how I exercised. Certain activities would have to be curtailed. I looked into my past and thought about what I would have to give up. I looked into the future, trying to figure out some way to adapt to this loss. Perhaps there was some less strenuous way I could exercise. . . . The ultrasound was normal. As quickly as I began this grief process, it was forgotten. I was able to return to a self-image of good health. Hence, it is not just dying that stimulates grief. Receiving a diagnosis of hypertension or diabetes can result in a grief reaction. As referred to elsewhere throughout this book, withdrawal of any care to which the patient and family have become accustomed can be experienced as grief. So, what is grief?

Grief is often experienced as a painful, tearing sensation, much like two strips of Velcro being pulled apart. The person's world has been ripped apart, opening a painful wound, which we call grief. However, grief is also a *process* wherein the grieving person works to create a new self in a new relationship with a changing world. Grief is a process of healing this wound. On one side of the wound is a self that has been torn from some object of attachment on the other side, the *loss-object*. Grief as a process can be understood as the adjustment to this radical change in the relationship between the self and the loss-object. Loss-objects may be people or something as simple as the pleasure of drinking coffee in the morning. The loss-object can even be one's own self-image. In the story of my possibly having a DVT, I was grieving an image of myself in a certain state of health. Grief can be understood as a process of physical, affective, and cognitive change that occurs in response to an abrupt alteration in the relationship between the grieving person and the loss-object. A central task in grieving is to redefine this relationship.[17] The grieving person moves, sometimes slowly, sometimes quickly, toward a new equilibrium as he or she redefines the relationship with the loss-object.

In considering this process, a paradox arises. Although the grieving person experiences a sense of separation or dislocation from the loss-object, in fact, the relationship *continues* between the grieving person and the loss-object. Grief as a process is not about completing a partial separation, like amputating a partially severed limb, but is about an evolving, changing, and ultimately new relationship between the self and the loss-object. Understanding this is critical to grief work. Bereaved individuals, if told that they must "get over" their grief, for example, may react by "freezing" their grief. They may fear that if they were to finish grieving by completing a psychic "amputation," they would truly lose their loved one forever. Many would prefer the pain of frozen grief to the prospect of such permanent loss. As bereaved people can readily tell you, they still have a relationship with the deceased; it just changes. My father died 10 years ago. I am still grieving this loss, albeit in a softer way. I will continue to have a relationship with my father as long as I have a self. Over the years this relationship has changed and will continue to change. Such continuity between the living and the dead is suggested in the following passage:

> Death is nothing at all. I have only slipped away into the next room. I am I and you are you. Whatever we were to each other, that we are still. Call me by my old familiar name, speak to me in the easy way you always use. Put no difference into your tone, wear no forced air of solemnity or sorrow. . . . What is death but negligible accident? Why should I be out of mind because I am out of sight? I am waiting for you, for an interval, somewhere very near just around the corner. All is well.
>   Henry Scott Holland (1847–1918), British Anglican clergyman

How does this process of grief occur? There is no simple answer. In complex ways, a new self evolves. One's self changes, as does one's image or understanding of the loss-object. In this process a new relationship is formed, and the wound heals. My grief for my father did not begin with his death, but with his growing infirmity and dependence well prior to his death. In the process of this grief I needed both to create a new self relative to my father, as a responsible adult son, and conversely to change my image of him from that of a powerful, independent father to one of a dependent father who needed care. It is a tribute to the human psyche that we can create new relationships in this way without destroying old ones.

Anticipatory (Preparatory) Grief

Preparatory grief is the grief "that the terminally ill patient has to undergo in order to prepare himself for his final separation from this world."[18]* Anticipatory grief occurs both in the dying and in those close to them.[19,20] Anticipatory grief is a normal grief reaction to perceived loss during the dying process. Dying people (and their loved ones) prepare for death by mourning the various losses implicit in the death. The anticipated loss of loved ones is obvious. The simple pleasures of living may also be grieved. The term *anticipatory* (or *preparatory*) *grief* is somewhat confusing. It is not as simple as preparing for a special event, such as a wedding, in the future. People are not preparing to grieve at some time in the future, they are grieving in the *present,* relative to a process of loss currently being experienced and projected into the future.

In facing death grieving people pay a great deal of attention to both the past and the future. In looking back, people often carefully examine themselves, the person(s) being lost, their relationships, their accomplishments, and their missed opportunities. It is as if they are reviewing a long story they have created, one full of heroes and villains, tragedy, comedy, and romance. How well was this story written? In this person's death, how will it end? If impending death is viewed as coming prematurely, part of the grief process can be thought of as a rewriting of this story.[21]

It seems most of us build our stories based on an optimistic story line in which we and our loved ones "live happily ever after." At some point, sometimes abruptly, sometimes gradually, this story line is challenged, with something like a "blank page" being introduced into the story.[22] Patients and families may initially experience chaos in response to this blank page. A normal response to such chaos is to try to reconstitute the original story line and to get back on track.[1] If reconstitution fails or is obviously impossible, then rewriting must begin anew. This rewriting does not begin on page one but must take up where the blank page has been introduced (although remembrance and interpretation of past events may change in light of the introduction of the blank page). Thus, people in grief engage in creating new story lines and new endings for stories begun years before. Major characters and their traits have been well defined. How they respond to this challenge of loss will be shaped by these traits. In this process hidden strengths and weaknesses may be exposed. The plot must be rewritten

*Kübler-Ross used the term *preparatory grief* explicitly in reference to the grief experienced by the dying person. Since then, the term *anticipatory grief* (or *anticipatory mourning* by Rando) has been more widely used and refers to grief and mourning before death for both patient and significant others.

to accommodate an ending in which everybody does not live happily ever after. This process of rewriting is the work of grief.

Bereavement

Bereavement is the grief that occurs after a death. Much has been written about bereavement grief.[20,23–28] In many ways bereavement has served as a model for understanding grief in other situations. Grief patterns in bereavement vary greatly among different cultures and individuals.[29] However, the essential processes of grief are similar. Waves of strong emotions, often triggered irregularly and unpredictably, wash up. In this process a new relationship is forged between the bereaved and the deceased, and over time these waves diminish in intensity.

The reader may wonder, why talk about bereavement in a text for clinicians, primarily physicians. In our medical culture we tend to see our relationships with the patient and family as ending with the death of the patient. Families often share this view. If bereavement is complicated (see below), this is best addressed by mental health workers. So why talk about bereavement?

There are three major reasons why the (non–mental health) clinician should be concerned about bereavement. First, the bereaved may have explicit needs that can be addressed only by a medical practitioner. Second, virtually everyone becomes bereaved at some point in life. How people cope in their bereavement can have a major effect on their health and health care decisions. You may not have cared for the person who died, but the bereaved spouse in your office who complains of insomnia or lack of appetite may be your patient. Finally, all clinicians need to be alert to signs that point to complicated bereavement so we can rally resources to help.

Questions for the medical practitioner

Bereaved individuals may have questions that only a medical practitioner can answer. Second thoughts may occur regarding treatment choices that were made. 'I can't help wondering, doctor, if we made the right choice when we decided to take George off life support. . . .' Having recovered from the shock phase of grief upon learning of the death of a loved one, some people may later need to come back to hear more explicitly the circumstances of the death. Autopsy results and their implications, both related to care that had been delivered and for future generations, may need to be discussed. These tasks cannot be relegated to counselors.

Bereavement as a health care risk factor

Recently bereaved people, especially geriatric patients, are at substantially higher risk for adverse events, including mortality. Parkes, in a study of 4486 widowers over the age of 55, found a 40% increased mortality rate compared to age-matched controls over six months.[30] Bereaved individuals may present with a variety of complaints, such as insomnia, anorexia, anxiety, and body pains, that may be manifestations of grief or grief that has transformed into clinical depression.[31] Some recently bereaved individuals may be concerned that they are "going crazy" if they see or hear the recently deceased. Rees interviewed 293 bereaved individuals and found that 47% had experienced such "hallucinations." The majority of those interviewed found such hallucinations (visual and auditory) helpful. Rees noted that, "It seems reasonable to conclude from theses studies that hallucinations are normal experiences after widowhood, providing helpful psychological phenomena to those experiencing them."[32] Thus, this phenomenon is not rare and can be considered to be within the normal range of grief reactions. People may need reassurance that these experiences are common and do not reflect psychosis. On the other hand, bereaved individuals may truly be unable to bear a loss and may suffer complicated grief reactions that require professional attention.

Complicated bereavement

Although grief in bereavement is itself a normal process, it can become complicated and harmful.[20,31,33] The best way to address complicated bereavement is to identify those individuals at high risk for it, work with them, if possible, before an anticipated death, and subsequently follow them closely. Unlike the healing process of normal bereavement, complicated bereavement is destructive to the individual. It results in dysfunctional behavior, poor quality of life, and, at times, even suicide. The more terrible the death and the more limited the coping abilities of the bereaved person, the greater is the risk of complicated bereavement. Violent or sudden deaths, deaths in which the bereaved may feel some sense of responsibility (such as the driver of a car in an auto accident), and deaths of young people result in a higher complicated bereavement risk.[25] Bereaved individuals who were highly dependent on the deceased, such as elderly spouses, are at higher risk, as are those who have earlier histories of mental illnesses. Poverty and cultural isolation also limit coping abilities. The clinician can be of great service in identifying such individuals as early as possible, because counseling and supportive services can be of immense help.

One hint of complicated bereavement to watch for is grief that appears to be frozen at a certain stage. In this case grief becomes less a process than a way of life. The parents of a child who died in an accident may preserve the child's room, like a shrine, for years following the death. The process of normal grief is not linear. Sometimes it proceeds very slowly and sometimes quickly. However, *no* change is worrisome. Individuals stuck in their grief generally benefit from counseling.

Working with Grieving Individuals

Although the clinician should know when to refer individuals with complicated grief, there is much they can do to address and facilitate grief when it arises. The acronym RELIEVER can serve as a reminder of simple interventions that anyone can do to assist the grieving, both in preparatory grief and bereavement.[7]

Reflect back emotions (mirroring and naming). Example: The person may say, "Why did I have to get this horrible disease." You might respond, "I can see that you are angry."

Empathize and make a personal connection. Example: "I can imagine that you are going through rough times. What can I do to help?"

Lead. Guided questions may help facilitate the grief process. Examples: "What concerns do you have about how your loved ones will do, after you are gone?" "When you went through difficult situations in the past, how did you handle them?"

Improvise. Respect emotional boundaries, and support individuals within those boundaries. The clinician's approach must be tailored to suit each individual. What may work with one person may fail with another. Some may desire support through talking, for example. Others may simply want your presence. Some may wish to have time alone, while others may cope best by continuing prior routines. Individuals may suddenly change coping strategies, which requires great flexibility in response by the clinician.

Educate. Explain that grief often comes in waves. Patients and families may need explanations of how others in the family can grieve in different ways. Recently bereaved individuals may need to be told that seeing or hearing the deceased occasionally does not mean they are going crazy.

Validate the Experience. Reflect back the normalcy of the experience. Example: "It is OK to cry," or "It seems to me you are responding normally to a very difficult situation."

Recall. Many grieving people need to look back over their lives. You may help the dying by asking them about their accomplishments, special stories, and legacies they wish to hand down to future generations. Bereaved individuals may benefit from telling stories about the good times they had with the deceased.

It is wonderful that the American Medicare hospice benefit requires bereavement support for the families of those who die in hospice. However, this has not become the standard of care for patients who die outside of hospice. This strikes me as terribly ironic. Relative to the other ways people die, hospice deaths tend to be the most peaceful and best anticipated. Support offered during the dying process probably reduces the risk of complicated bereavement in survivors. For those deaths that are most likely to result in complex bereavement—violent deaths and the deaths of young people in hospitals—no support is considered necessary, and often none is given (unless mass death occurs, as in an airplane crash or school shooting). This simply does not make sense. I suspect this results from a narrow interpretation of who the patient is and what our roles should be; according to this way of thinking, when the patient dies, the relationship between the clinician and the family ends because the patient's life has ended. Obviously, things are not so simple. It is probable that family members are also patients of our health care system and, as discussed above, bereavement is a health care risk factor for morbidity and mortality. Beyond this, it seems to me that some minimum degree of bereavement follow-up is simply the right, humane thing to do.

Establishing a comprehensive bereavement support system for the dying may not be politically feasible at the current time. However, I believe we could take one small step in the right direction. I hope that someday each hospital and each health care system will establish a policy such that if and when somebody dies in the hospital, someone will attempt to make one telephone call offering condolences on behalf of the hospital. This would not break the bank. It is only a tiny gesture. Who can argue that we should not call the parent of a child brought to the ER who was killed by a truck or the spouse of a man who died on the operating table? Is one phone call too much to ask? It is my hope that someday this will become a minimum standard of care.

Altered States of Consciousness at the End of Life

Fred was a librarian who was shy and obsessive about details. Unfortunately, he developed a glioblastoma multiforme, a brain tumor from which he was dying. Fred's wife, Hanna, in contrast, was an extrovert who was florid in dress and personality. They were a classic odd couple. When Fred came to us, he had become bedridden. As with most patients with brain tumors, he had little pain. His suffering arose from progressive disorientation that resulted from his growing tumor. Self-control had always been important to Fred, and he found it intolerable that he did not understand exactly what was going on. He grumbled and complained. One day close to the end of his life when I went to see him, I sensed something different. The struggle for control had faded. He sighed, "I just wish I could get away. To a . . . South Sea island. But I know I can't." I cannot say exactly how I knew, but I understood that this was no ordinary conversation. Fred was in an altered state. I sensed an important opening. "Well," I said, let's go. Let's hop on the plane and fly off to Tahiti." "Really?" His face came alive with the possibility. "We can go?" "Sure, I said. I've got two tickets right here." For a moment his face lit up. Then a shadow fell. "Oh no," he said, "there is just no way I can go." He looked like he might cry. "Why not," I asked, puzzled. "Look at all this," he said, pointing around the bed. "Look at all this luggage. I'll never get on the plane." "Shoot, what are we going to need luggage for," I replied. "We're just going to be lying on the beach, sipping margaritas." With that, I hopped onto his bed, and he and I began chucking luggage out of the "plane" as he laughed and laughed. Hanna stood in the doorway with tears running down her cheeks. As I passed by, she said, "I've waited 20 years for him to get rid of that goddamn luggage." Fred died a few days later.

Dying patients frequently experience altered states of consciousness toward the end of life. Unfortunately, the vocabulary we have to discuss such states is limited. *Delirium* is a word often used. However, the word *delirium* has a completely negative connotation, whereas some altered states are pleasant, even ecstatic.[34] Altered states, as in Fred's case, can even hold the potential for growth. Here, I attempt to provide a framework for the consideration of altered states in a less biased manner, leaving open the possibility that not all altered states are bad. Sadly, the evidence base for much of this discussion is poor. I hope that future studies can critically examine what is proposed here.

It is very difficult to state the prevalence of altered states of consciousness at the end of life. Studies that used various terminologies and methodologies cite rates from 25% to 85%.[9,35–38] Clearly, altered states of varying degree and quality are not rare. Helping patients who experience these altered states and their families can be extremely challenging.

Altered states are nothing unusual in and of themselves. Whenever we dream we experience an "altered state," compared to wakeful consciousness. We have come to accept this as normal. In dying patients at certain times altered states may also be normal. As we shall see, the issue often is not so much what is "normal" as whether suffering is associated with the altered state.

I have found these factors useful in analyzing altered states—the level of consciousness, orientation (or wavelength), and the content of the altered state.

Level of Consciousness

The level of consciousness may be decreased, increased, or roughly the same as that experienced in normal wakefulness. At one extreme, comatose patients have very low levels of consciousness. At the other extreme, agitated patients have a "higher" level of consciousness (or alertness). Most patients who have an increased level of consciousness that I have treated experience some distress. However, a patient may rarely experience a heightened level of consciousness as an ecstatic moment, as did Fred while chucking the luggage. Levels of consciousness often fluctuate rapidly in patients who have altered states.

What is the effect of a certain level of consciousness on a particular patient? A lower level of consciousness, being sleepy, may be highly desirable for some and seems to be in tune with the dying process. For others this can be very distressing. Others may wish to be sleepy and may become disturbed when they are alert and awake.

Orientation

Physicians are usually taught to assess orientation to time, place, person, and situation (orientation × 4). This is a reasonable but crude way of thinking of orientation. Most useful in assessing altered states is orientation to *time*. The best single screening question to assess orientation related to altered states and delirium in a patient may be, "What time of day is it." Asking about date and year, a more commonly asked question by physicians, mixes *orientation* with *memory* of time. This is a good screening question for dementia but less useful for altered states or delirium. Most people know *who* they are deep into altered states. *Person* is more likely to be forgotten with severe memory loss, as in dementia. *Place* and *situation* are the most significant criteria in assessing orientation. It is important to distinguish between what is remembered or forgotten (possible dementia) compared to what is being experienced (possible altered state). A demented patient may forget being admitted to a hospital (place) for treatment of pneumonia (situation) and not be in an altered state. However, if a patient so admitted reports that he or she is on a cruise ship in the Bahamas, that is a very different experience, an altered state, whether the patient is demented or not.

Palliative Care Note

The most useful screening question for assessing altered states may be, "What time of day is it?"

I find it useful in considering this aspect of orientation to think by analogy about radio frequencies. In normal wakefulness we function and interact on a relatively narrow and shared frequency that allows both transmission and reception of shared experiences. When patients at the end of life experience altered states, it is as if their radio frequency, their wavelength, has shifted. Sometimes the dial is only slightly turned, which allows the patient to experience both the "normal" wavelength on which we coexist and yet receive signals on a wavelength that we cannot perceive. Such a patient might be perfectly aware of being in a hospital bed and of dying but be able to see and hear a deceased relative sitting in a chair next to the bed. Fred, the librarian, was on such a mixed frequency, which allowed me some access to his altered state experience. Sometimes the radio dial is turned farther, so that the patient becomes oblivious to our wavelength and experiences something completely different. Our only clues to such shifts are either the patient speaking or gesturing in an indicative way or the patient reporting on the experience after returning to our wavelength.

At this point I must stress that in discussing such altered states, I am not commenting on whether the late Aunt Edna is really sitting next to the dying patient, that is, whether such altered states are *real*. The point is they are *experienced* as real. This shifting of wavelengths may seem fantastic, but, in fact, we experience such states every night when we dream. Most of the time the shift is complete. When we dream, we experience a very different reality. However, sometimes we get caught in-between. Half-awake, half-asleep, our experience is a blend of different wavelengths. Such blending is very common in the dying, who appear to be "letting go" of a very rigid separation between daytime wakefulness and nighttime dreaming. This can be distressing to both patients and family members if it is not understood. Educating the patient and family can help normalize this experience. Frequently, I do so by drawing an analogy to dreaming, which people generally understand and find less threatening than speaking about hallucinations or the patient "going crazy."

Palliative Care Note

Comparing altered states to dreaming (rather than "going crazy") can help normalize such states and provide a frame of reference for patient and family understanding.

Content

For most patients in advanced stages of dying, content is the real issue, not level of consciousness or orientation. What is it that is being experienced? Is it pleasant or unpleasant, ecstatic or hellish? How can we help when suffering occurs that results from unpleasant content?

In analyzing the content of certain altered states at the end of life, we begin to appreciate how different it is from delirium as it is usually discussed in geriatrics and psychiatry. *Toxic* delirium, the type usually discussed by geriatricians and psychiatrists, is usually an unpleasant experience. The level of consciousness often fluctuates. The visual content of the experience is often very simple, for example, neon-green ants going up the wall or purple snakes under the bed—repetitive patterns often in psychedelic colors. I suspect such patterns result, in some way, from a deranged neuroexcitory state, perhaps one that enhances similar patterns that we see when our eyes are closed. I call this state a toxic delirium because in my experience there is usually a correctable, toxic cause. The delirium usually resolves when the cause is addressed. These patterns are commonly imposed on an otherwise normal experience; the ants or snakes are seen in a *hospital* room, not on a cruise ship.

Altered states at the end of life, if not associated with toxic delirium, most closely resemble dream states. Although levels of consciousness may vary, they can also be entirely normal. When there is overlap of wavelengths between waking reality and altered states, the introduced content is very different from that of toxic delirium. It usually involves people and a story (often relating to travel, as in Fred's case). Some have called these experiences "pre-death visions."[39] Most commonly seen are deceased relatives. It is remarkable how frequent an occurrence this is—estimated to occur before at least 25% of deaths. Also remarkable is the fact that virtually always the relatives are, in fact, dead; visits by otherwise unseen living relatives are rare. Next most frequent, in my experience, are guardian beings, angels and others. These beings (and often deceased relatives) seem to act as guardians of a barrier. Often, they will communicate to the patient that their time (to die, to cross-over) has not yet come or some similar message. I have noticed no correlation between the appearance of such beings and religiosity in patients. Usually, such angelic visitors are welcomed, although frustration may be experienced in not being allowed to complete the journey, join the group, or cross-over. (George, a devout atheist patient of mine, was an exception to this rule. When angels appeared in his room, he screamed, "Get out of here, there is no God!") Finally, other beings who are unknown to the patient will occasionally appear, most frequently children. In my experience, unlike the adults, the children are usually unknown to the patient and usually do not speak. They may walk in front of the patient's room or sleep at the foot of the bed or in a chair. Only rarely are the visits of such beings disturbing to the patient.

The one disease process I know of that can mimic these predeath visions is Parkinson's disease, especially when associated with Lewy bodies dementia.[40] These patients also have visual hallucinations, usually of people. The distinction is that usually the people in visions are unknown to the patient. Initially, the Parkinson patient may be aware that these people are not real; they may be only shadow figures. When turned to, they disappear. As the disease progresses, the patient usually becomes more paranoid and very disturbed by more persistent and troublesome visitations. Rare as Lewy bodies dementia is (a misnomer, in my opinion, as memory loss is not usually so prominent as is the fluctuating altered state), this disease is near to my heart because my mother suffered greatly with and died from this terrible illness.

In advanced stages of dying, when there is a more dramatic shifting of wavelengths, the entire experience of the patient can change in a dreamlike fashion. Frequently, past life events are relived. Life dramas may be worked out in metaphorical form, as happened in Fred's case. If the content of the experience is pleasant and lacks suffering, direct intervention is unnecessary. Explanation and coaching of the family is often required to explain that such states are common and that as long as the experience is pleasant, no treatment is needed. Family members may themselves be distressed and experience a grief reaction as they now feel disconnected from the dying person. If the patient becomes distressed because of disturbed content, then further evaluation and treatment is required.

Evaluation and Treatment of Altered States

Patients (and families) may experience distress related to altered levels of consciousness, orientation, and content. Patients may be seen as too alert, too sleepy, or unresponsive. Patients who are aware they are experiencing altered states may become distressed by the change in orientation. However, the greatest cause of distress usually relates to content—*what* the patient is experiencing. If that experience is distressing, we can reasonably call it *delirium*. A variety of screening tools have been developed for the detection of delirium.[41] As demonstrated by Grassi and colleagues, the commonly used mini-mental status examination (MMSE) has a high sensitivity (96%) but a low specificity (38%) for delirium.[42] Thus, this test is useful for ruling out delirium, but low (positive) scores may represent false positives.

The clinician should consider whether the nature of the delirium is suggestive of a *toxic* or a *terminal* delirium. An acute onset of delirium in a patient who does not appear to be very close to death is more suggestive of a toxic delirium. My impression is that toxic deliriums are much more amenable to treatment than are terminal deliriums. Lawlor, in a prospective study of 104 cancer patients treated on a palliative care ward, found a reversible cause 49% of the time in 71 patients who developed delirium.[43] (A clinical distinction between toxic and terminal delirium was not made in this study.) Suspicion of a toxic delirium should prompt a search for a correctable cause unless the patient is very close to death. Medications should be reviewed and adjusted as necessary. Consideration should be given to checking electrolytes, in particular sodium and calcium (with albumin). As Lawlor's group demonstrated, delirium may respond to a course of hydration. Both toxic and terminal delirium may be exacerbated by physical symptoms that have gone unrecognized or are undertreated. If patients are verbal, physical pain and other symptoms may be reinterpreted and reported in other terms. A painful rib metastasis may become a devil poking the patient in the side. Often, one must quietly observe the patient for some time to get a clue as to the underlying cause of distress. I recall one woman who was moaning and thrashing in her bed. Occasionally her hand moved to her groin, the only clue to her urinary retention. Catheter placement resolved the distress. Sometimes the disturbed content reflects some unresolved psychological issue or unpleasant memory. For example, one patient of mine with a somewhat shady past was in an altered state when he was "visited" by some old friends. When I asked if he was enjoying the visit, he replied, "Nope, 'cause I owe them money." He was playing cards with his "friends"—a metaphorical, dreamlike way of settling old scores.

Treatment of Terminal Delirium

Sadly, many clinicians have been poorly trained in this area and cannot distinguish among toxic delirium, terminal delirium, and normal altered states. Clinicians may not recognize that the patient is, in fact, dying. To approach altered states using the standard algorithm for toxic delirium can have disastrous consequences. Medications are reviewed for those that might cause delirium. Often, such medications are then withheld. In toxic delirium, such an approach often results in clinical improvement. Most dying patients I see are on opioids for pain and really need them. Sudden cessation of opioids results in chemical withdrawal and pain exacerbation that usually worsens the patient's delirium content. A new devil with a pitchfork may then appear.

While good studies are lacking, a number of experts in the field have commented that one of the factors that distinguishes terminal from nonterminal (toxic) delirium is that terminal delirium may not improve with standard therapy, such as medication withdrawal and the administration of neuroleptics.[44,45] That is, disorientation continues, although it may be improved in mild cases. Pharmacologic treatment revolves around a central question: is the goal of therapy to reorient the patient or sedate the patient? Standard therapy for delirium focuses almost exclusively on the first goal, reorientation. For refractory distress, reorientation simply does not work in advanced stages of dying. Sedation is frequently the only available pharmacologic option. Breitbart estimates that this is necessary in one-third of cases.[45]

Reorientation

Mild cases may respond to medications such as haloperidol (or newer neuroleptics such as risperidone and olanzapine) and result in improved orientation. However, severe disorientation associated with distress rarely returns to normal. Haloperidol can be given either as a standing order or as an as-needed medication with upward titration as appropriate. It is important to understand that haloperidol has minimal sedating effects. If patients become less agitated, it is usually because they are better oriented. Haloperidol has been found to be particularly useful for patients with disorientation at night (sundowning), as in dementia. Patients with Parkinson's disease cannot tolerate haloperidol. Risperidone or olanzapine may be used in its stead. Psychiatrists may assist with the dosing of these agents.

Sedation

The decision to sedate a patient should never be undertaken lightly.[46] A sedated patient will be less able to interact with his or her environment. If the patient is still eating and drinking, sedation strong enough to interfere with these functions becomes ethically problematic.[47] Fortunately, in most cases that require strong sedation, the patient has already stopped eating and drinking, which minimizes concern that the sedating process might hasten death. The decision to employ sedation should follow discussion with the patient, when clear (if possible), and/or the patient's proxy. Documentation of patient and/or proxy involvement in the decision to sedate should be included in the medical record. Having said this, it is important to recognize that sedation occurs along a wide spectrum, from very low doses of lorazepam, for example, at one end to rare cases using general anesthesia at the other. Most patients require only small to modest doses of sedating agents titrated not to coma, but to peaceful drowsiness. Deep sedation (variously called terminal, total, or palliative sedation) should be reserved for patients with otherwise intractable distress who are very close to death. In all cases the physician must weigh the potential benefits and burdens of sedation. To avoid any possible misunderstandings as to the intent of such sedation, orders and medical record documentation should be as explicit as possible regarding the endpoint(s) against which the sedating dose is to be titrated. For example, the order may read, "drug X given PRN qY hours for distress as evidenced by grimacing, moaning, or statements of pain or suffering." When the agreed-upon endpoint has been reached, further upward titration ceases, and the drug dose is stabilized.

A variety of sedatives may be used.[9,38,48] Benzodiazepines, such as lorazepam, can be sedating, although some care must be used, particularly in the elderly, because they may cause further disorientation and disinhibit the patient.[44,49] Rather like one drink of alcohol, 0.5 mg of lorazepam may make some people sleepy while disinhibiting others, resulting in wild behavior. Higher doses of lorazepam may be needed for sedation. Anticholinergic agents such as scopolamine, commonly given for respiratory secretions in those who are actively dying, may also produce adequate sedation.

Sedating neuroleptics, such as chlorpromazine and thioridazine, are commonly employed in hospice. I have had the most experience with chlorpromazine. Chlorpromazine has the advantage of coming in a very concentrated oral solution, 100 mg/cc. Often 10–20 mg (0.1–.2 cc) will adequately sedate, and it can be administered orally even to patients unable to swallow. Chlorpromazine can also be given via rectal suppositories, IM, but not SC and only rarely in a diluted

IV solution. Chlorpromazine blocks dopamine, cholinergic, and histaminic receptors as well as alpha receptors. It should be avoided in patients with Parkinson's disease and in patients prone to orthostatic hypotension. Chlorpromazine (and other neuroleptics) can lower the seizure threshold. It should not be used in patients with active seizure disorders and only with caution in those prone to seizures. It is virtually impossible to predict a therapeutic dose. Some patients respond to very low doses, and some require considerably higher doses. In severely agitated patients doses should be given every hour, gradually increasing the dosage until the desired clinical end-point (lack of evidence of distress) is obtained. Based on the amount of drug given, the patient can be maintained on q6–q8-hour dosing.

When chlorpromazine is contraindicated or ineffective, barbiturates may be given. They have an additional advantage of being anticonvulsants in patients with seizures. Again, proper dosing must be individualized. I have found phenobarbital elixir useful. Phenobarbital has a slow onset and prolonged action. Pentobarbital (Nembutal) is faster in onset and can be given via rectal suppositories. Pentobarbital can also be given IM. Dosing intervals for the patient should be individualized because of a highly variable plasma half-life. Rarely, short-acting sedatives such as midazolam or propofol may be required for sedation of severely agitated patients when quick titration is desired. Consultation from either palliative care experts or anesthesiologists should first be obtained.

Nonpharmacologic Interventions

In most cases nonpharmacologic interventions should be used in conjunction with pharmacologic interventions. Patients in distressed altered states at the end of life can be remarkably sensitive to their environments. Maintaining a peaceful, quiet environment is essential. Family members and staff should be coached, if necessary, to speak lovingly to the patient and to encourage pleasant aspects of the experience while carefully steering patients away from unpleasant content. This is what I attempted to do with Fred, the librarian. Working with patients in distressed altered states is difficult and requires experience to do so well. Although specific guidelines are beyond the scope of this book, a few principles can be shared.

Some mildly disoriented patients can be reoriented through simple interventions—open windows (revealing day and night), clocks, and straightforward reminders of what is happening. Some patients cannot be so oriented and may become distressed by attempts to do so. In such cases recall that for the person experiencing an altered state, it is *real*. Going along and guiding the patient through such a state is not the same as humoring the patient. The altered experience must be approached respectfully. Suggestions to encourage positive aspects of the experience may be given, and the patient may be distracted or diverted from negative aspects. The presence of loving family members and their peaceful words and soothing touches can go far toward encouraging a positive experience. Sometimes, the best thing to do is back off for a while and use time as your ally. For example, rather than force an agitated patient to take a bath, wait until the agitation (bad dream) passes. Returning later, you may find the patient much more amenable to what you suggest. (This principle may also work well with patients suffering from dementia, who may resist some care, such as a bath, but then forget why they resisted and agree a short time later.)

The Potential for Growth

The possibility of personal growth in the dying process is a central tenet of the hospice movement. Such growth may occur despite or because of suffering. Not all growth requires normal orientation. In fact, my experience tells me that altered states are necessary for growth in certain people, as I believe was the case for Fred, the librarian. Only then are certain deeper truths revealed.

I end this section on altered states with an additional brief story. One day while on rounds I came upon Mr. R. He was sitting up in bed with his eyes closed and a half-smile on his face. In front of him was a stand with some flowers on it. "Are you resting?" I asked. "No," he replied, "meditating." He told me he was in his garden looking at the flowers. He was not "imagining" this garden, he was there. I asked, "Do you see that one flower?" He nodded yes, and I could sense that his mind was coming into focus. He said, "A perfect rose. No beginning or end. Nothing more to say." With that we parted, and for me this became his death poem, as he died shortly thereafter. I am grateful for the gift of his wisdom in this most wonderful of poems.

Spirituality

"Do you believe in God?" "What do you think will happen to us when we die?" "Why did God do this to me?" "Doctor, will you pray for me?" Some would say that the clinician has no business dealing with spirituality or religion. How, then, should we answer questions such as these? Whatever our beliefs about the nature of the universe and our roles as clinicians, we cannot escape the fact that for many of our patients and their families, spirituality (or religion) is central to their lives and becomes particularly important as they approach death.[50,51] If we are to be of some assistance, we must deal with people as they are, and this means we have no choice but to deal with the spiritual aspects of their experience. Studies have suggested that many patients want, but rarely receive, physician involvement in their spiritual care. King, for example, studied 203 adult inpatients and found that 77% of those surveyed thought that physicians should consider patients' spiritual needs; 37% wanted physicians to discuss religious beliefs more frequently. However, 68% reported that physicians had never discussed religious beliefs.[52]

Spirituality is that aspect of a person's beliefs and experience that *transcends* the everyday world. Religion is an organized belief system. These may be my definitions, but what matters more is what they mean to our patients and their families. Some may reject both terms outright: "I have no beliefs," or "I'm an atheist." Fine; these, too, are beliefs that arise from a certain understanding of what makes the universe tick. What is *meaningful* to such a person? How does such a perspective affect that individual's understanding of his or her living and dying? Where is suffering to be found, and where solace? The danger in working with people who express "no beliefs" is in taking such statements at face value. Questions of meaning, suffering, and solace are still highly relevant and, in the broadest sense, are also spiritual.[53]

Some will take offense at the term *spirituality*, thinking this refers to some cultlike belief system. "I'm a born-again Christian." "I'm Jewish" (or "Buddhist," or whatever). Fine; what does that *mean* to you? We are burdened in such exchanges by preconceptions. We may know something about Christianity, Judaism, or Buddhism, and therefore we may think we know something about what it means to this person. Very often we are wrong. The same questions arise: what is meaningful to you, where is your suffering, where is your solace? And how can we help you in all this?

Is this not a job for a chaplain or spiritual care adviser? Certainly. As elsewhere in medicine, clinicians need to know when to refer to others for help. However, not everything can be referred. If a patient asks you, "Doctor, why did this happen to me," or "Doctor, what is your faith," how will you answer? Charles von Gunten, chair of the American Board of Hospice and Palliative Medicine, is fond of saying that "why" questions that do not rely on technical explanations are spiritual in nature. You may choose to answer, "You got cancer because you smoked four packs a day," but is this what the patient is really asking? When asked about your faith, you may begin a lecture on your beliefs or lack thereof, but is this really what the patient needs?

Palliative Care Note

"Why" questions that do not depend upon technical answers are often spiritual in nature—Charles von Gunten.*

---

*Personal statement. Dr. Charles von Gunten is the current chair of the American Board of Hospice and Palliative Medicine and is coprincipal investigator for the EPEC (Education for Physicians on End-of-Life Care). He is also a dear friend.

It may seem strange, but an important starting point in addressing spirituality relates to skill training. Spirituality is complex and profound. All of us in some way, I think, are struggling to make sense of this universe. Rather than take on the heaviest of issues, it is better to start with babysteps. Later, we may contemplate the deep inner meaning of it all.

FICA—A Spiritual Assessment Tool*

Christina Pulchalski has developed an acronym, FICA, which can be used in performing a spiritual assessment:[55,56]

Faith: "What do you believe in that gives meaning to your life?" A broad, open-ended question is usually asked. There is no single correct question, although Dr. Pulchalski has found the above and the following to be useful. "Do you consider yourself to be a religious or spiritual person?" Both *religious* and *spiritual* are used because individuals may relate to one and may even take offense at the other. Many individuals who will say they are not religious will admit to being spiritual, which should prompt a discussion of what this means to them. Conversely, an answer such as, "Yes, I'm Catholic," tells you something but begs exploration of what this means.

Importance and Influence: "How important is your faith (or religion or spirituality) to you?" Just hearing that the person is spiritual or a member of a particular religion tells you little. How *important* is this? *How* is it important? There is a big difference between a Catholic who has not been to Mass since childhood and one who goes to Mass daily.

Community: "Are you a part of a religious or spiritual community?" Particularly for those who participate in organized religion, community is often a central part of their spiritual and social experience. It is not uncommon that just when this community becomes most important, when death approaches, the individual is cut off from that community because of illness and care-giving needs.

Address or Application: "How would you like me to address these issues in your health care?" "How might these things apply to your current situation?" "How can we assist you in your spiritual care?" Patients and families often feel better simply because they have been given permission to share their beliefs. That you have inquired is usually seen as a sign of respect. However, there may be very specific things you can do to be of assistance. In a talk on

*See Fast Fact #19, Taking a Spiritual History, for an alternative acronym, SPIRIT: S. Spiritual belief system, P personal spirituality, I Integration with a spiritual community, R Ritualized practice and restrictions, I Implications for medical care, T terminal event planning.[54] Ambuel B. and D. E. Weissman, *Fast Fact and Concept #19; Taking a Spiritual History*. 1999, End of Life Education Project: http://www.eperc.mcw.edu/.

assessing suffering, Baines told the story of a man who reported 10 of 10 on a scale of suffering that related entirely to his spiritual care. He had regularly attended a certain service and was now unable to do so, which resulted in unbearable suffering. With permission the hospice team contacted the ministry, which sent a home ministry team to the patient's home. His suffering score drop to 0 of 10.[57] As in this case, *assistance* for many will mean *access*. A simple phone call to the proper clergy member can significantly relieve distress. Patients and families may also have fears related to spiritual issues that they may be hesitant to express. For example, Sikhs wear sacred regalia that should not be removed from the person at any time.[58] Patients and families may become terrified that health care workers will remove them. Asking if patients have any special concerns or fears and then addressing them may be of great assistance.

Like all mnemonics, FICA has a certain artificiality. Dr. Pulchalski has stressed that performing it usually takes only a few minutes and can reveal a wealth of information. She also points out that it often leads naturally to other discussions, such as an exploration of patient and family preferences. Such discussions often make more sense following an exploration of spirituality. It is also possible to incorporate aspects of FICA into the normal flow of conversation. In my experience many patients and families toss out a hint that they would like to enter a discussion of spirituality with a statement such as, "Why do you think this happened to me?" The clinician faces a choice—cut off that thread with a response such as, "Darned if I know," or expand the lead by saying "I wish I knew. What do you think?" Most people do not expect us to have the answers. However, they are looking for an opportunity to share and explore their own beliefs and concerns. The clinician may reflect back such questions: "Why do you think this has happened to you?" Such reflection often naturally leads to a broader exploration of spirituality.

It has puzzled me that so little work, even in palliative care, has gone into teaching clinicians about dealing with spirituality. Even the American Medical Association EPEC (Educating Physicians about End-of-Life Care) program did not include a module on this. When we first attempted to include spirituality as a topic in our End-of-Life Care (ELC) faculty development curriculum at the Stanford Faculty Development Center, we got a clearer sense of why this might be so. Not surprisingly (in retrospect), the physicians we were training had strong opinions about spirituality. Some physicians seemed to be just waiting for the opportunity to bring spirituality to the fore. Although we tried to stress that the focus in raising spirituality as a topic area was on what spirituality means to the patient and family and that our curriculum should be useful to *all* physicians, including atheists, some participants seemed unable to resist the temptation of making strong statements regarding their own beliefs. One student began a practice session on spirituality by stating, "You are all spiritual beings"—or words to that effect, which made some cringe. Although I might personally agree with such a statement, I think it is very important that any clinician training in this area be assiduously neutral relative to the importance, or *value*, of spirituality apart from the value spirituality holds for our patients and families. Not to do so risks an imposition of beliefs and values that many quite rightly would find offensive. Not everybody agrees that "We are all spiritual beings."

We remain committed to discussing spirituality as a component of our curriculum but have learned that a special cautionary note is called for. To put it bluntly, it is not about you, it is about the patient and family. In teaching spirituality as a component of a broader palliative care curriculum, it is not what I, the teacher, believes or you, the learner, believes that is most important. It is about acquiring skills necessary to address the spiritual needs of patients and families, period. If spirituality is important to you in your life and your work (as it personally is in mine), fine—let your spirituality shine through the quality of care you deliver and the quality of your teaching. Sometimes, when a patient asks "Do you believe in God," he or she really is curious about how you are struggling with this issue as a person. Sharing your thoughts and beliefs *may* meet a need of the patient to know that we physicians, too, are mortal and are struggling with the same big questions. Most patients and families are relatively preoccupied with their own struggle and ask such questions as an inquiry to determine if you are open to exploring *their* spiritual concerns. I might say something such as "I'm still struggling myself to understand what this world is all about. What about you? What do *you* believe?"

Each Person Dies His or Her Own Death

Of course, how could it be otherwise. Nevertheless, people try to impose their notions of a good death on the dying all the time. All of us have some idea of what it would mean to die well.[59-62] For some, dying well is not "spiritual" at all. It is about pain control and, perhaps, taking care of business, such as wills and funeral arrangements. For many it is about relationships—asking forgiveness, being forgiven, expressing one's love and thanks, and saying goodbye. For others, dying well means an essential preparation for an afterlife with eternal consequences. If one believes that he or she will spend all eternity in hell if certain things are not accomplished, the stakes are very high indeed.

It can be very difficult to accept that others choose to live and die in a manner that we may judge to be foolish or harmful. It can be very difficult for me, personally, when I see a dying person or family approach death in a manner that seems to actively generate suffering. I have to remind myself that my job is not to fix, not to eliminate, suffering, but to *alleviate* it. Well-intentioned interventions may be declined. This saddens me, but it must be so. Sometimes, I am angered by the misery patients and families seem to heap upon themselves. I think, "Can't they see what they are doing, the fools?" Sometimes, I have to remind myself that *dying* is part of *living* and that, just as people have every right to be "fools" in everyday life (in my very biased view), so they do in dying. What makes it difficult for me, I think, is that if people are "foolish" in everyday life, it is relatively easy to ignore them. However, the dying and their families depend on us for care. Their suffering is all too visible, even palpable. We cannot walk away. To the extent we can empathize, we, too, will suffer. One of the hardest things in palliative care is to maintain a passion and commitment to good care balanced by a certain detachment—to do the work for the *doing* without getting hung up on the outcome. Not everybody wants what we have to offer. Not everybody has the same idea as to what constitutes a good death or a good life.

People who choose palliative care as a profession tend to be incorrigible do-gooders. We like to see people who are suffering healed by our hands. Many of us also thrive on the praise and adulation we receive from patients and families for our work. Thus, if patients or families choose a different path and spurn our efforts at healing, or if we are criticized, we tend to take it hard and personally. When this happens to me, I try to remind myself, again and again, that it is not about me, it is about our patients and families. We are not in charge of the outcomes. This is not some symphony we are conducting; we are just there to try to help, to lend a hand. That some will accept our help and some not, that some peoples' dying will seem easier than that of others, is just the way it goes.

Although this material could have been written in any part of this book, I chose to include it here, as our spiritual beliefs and biases tend to run deep. As we come to understand how much suffering relates to spiritual distress, it is tempting to share our own beliefs and practices with those who suffer. However, my impression is that most people are remarkably immune to spiritual imposition. Most of us, I think, would resent the imposition of a form of alien spirituality. It does not work, and it is irritating. This does not mean, however, that our own spirituality cannot serve us. To the extent spirituality is important to us as clinicians, I believe it can invest every aspect of our work. How you feel a pulse or perform a rectal examination will say more about your spiritual practice than will any philosophical comments you might make on the meaning of life and death.

References

1. Frank, A. *The Wounded Storyteller—Body, Illness, and Ethics.* 1995, University of Chicago Press: Chicago, pp. 75–114.
2. Block, S. D. Assessing and managing depression in the terminally ill patient. ACP-ASIM End-of-Life Care Consensus Panel. American College of Physicians—American Society of Internal Medicine. Ann Intern Med 2000; 132(3): 209–18.

3. Periyakoil, V. and D. E. Weissman. Fast Fact and Concept #43: Is it grief or depression? End of Life Education Project. http://www.eperc.mcw.edu/, 2001.
4. McDowell, I. and C. Newell. *Measuring Health*, 2nd ed. 1996, Oxford University Press: New York, pp. 259–63.
5. Chochinov, H. M. et al. "Are you depressed?" Screening for depression in the terminally ill. Am J Psychiatry 1997; 154(5): 674–6.
6. Porter, M. et al. From sadness to major depression: Assessment and management in patients with cancer. In: R.K. Portenoy and E. Bruera, eds. *Topics in Palliative Care*. 1998, Oxford University Press: New York, pp. 191–212.
7. Periyakoil, V. S. and J. Hallenbeck. Identifying and managing preparatory grief and depression at the end of life. Am Fam Physician 2002; 65(5): 883–90.
8. Breitbart, W. and P. Jacobsen. Psychiatric symptoms in management in terminal care. Clin Geriatr Med 1996; 12: 329–47.
9. Breitbart, W., H. M. Chochinov, et al. Psychiatric aspects of palliative care. In: D. Doyle, G. Hanks, et al. *The Oxford Textbook of Palliative Medicine*. 1998, Oxford University Press: New York, pp. 934–54.
10. Homsi, J., D. Walsh, et al. Psychostimulants in supportive care. Support Care Cancer 2000; 8(5): 385–97.
11. von Molke, L., D. Greenblatt, et al. Clinical pharmacokinetics of antidepressants in the elderly; Therapeutic implications. Clin Pharmacokinet 1993; (24): 141–60.
12. Miller, L. J. Gabapentin for treatment of behavioral and psychological symptoms of dementia. Ann Pharmacother 2001; 35(4): 427–31.
13. Pande, A. C. et al. Placebo-controlled study of gabapentin treatment of panic disorder. J Clin Psychopharmacol 2000; 20(4): 467–71.
14. Kast, R. E. Mirtazapine may be useful in treating nausea and insomnia of cancer chemotherapy. Support Care Cancer 2001; 9(6): 469–70.
15. Goodnick, P. J. et al. Mirtazapine in major depression with comorbid generalized anxiety disorder. J Clin Psychiatry 1999; 60(7): 446–8.
16. Hallenbeck, J. and D. E. Weissman. Fast Fact and Concept #33; Grief and bereavement. End of Life Education Project. http://www.eperc.mcw.edu/, 2001.
17. Worden, J. *Grief Counseling and Grief Therapy*, 2nd ed. 1991, Springer: New York.
18. Kübler-Ross, E. *On Death and Dying*. 1969, Macmillan: New York.
19. Zilberfein, F. *Coping with death: Anticipatory grief and bereavement*. GENERATIONS/Care at the End-of-Life: Restoring a Balance 1999(Spring,): 69–74.
20. Katz, L. and K. Chocinov. The spectrum of grief in palliative care. In: R.K. Portenoy and E. Bruera, eds. *Topics in Palliative Care*. 1998, Oxford University Press: New York, pp. 295–310.
21. Becker, G. *Disrupted Lives—How People Create Meaning in a Chaotic World*. 1999, University of California Press: Berkeley.
22. Good, B. *Medicine, Rationality, and Experience: An Anthropological Perspective*. 1994, Cambridge University Press: New York, pp. 66–184.
23. Schoenberg, G. et al., eds. *Bereavement—Its Psychosocial Aspects*. 1975, Columbia University Press: New York.
24. Rando, T. *Grief, Dying and Death. Clinical Interventions for Caregivers*. 1984, Research Press: Champaign, Ill.
25. Doka, K., ed. *Living with Grief after Sudden Loss*. 1996, Hospice Foundation of America: Washington, D.C.
26. Doka, K., ed. *Living with Grief: Children, Adolescents, and Loss*. 2000, Hospice Foundation of America: Washington, D.C.

27. *The pediatrician and childhood bereavement. American Academy of Pediatrics Committee on Psychosocial Aspects of Child and Family Health.* Pediatrics 2000; 105(2): 445–7.

28. Worden, J. W. Bereavement care. In: A. Berger, ed. *Principles and Practice of Supportive Oncology.* 1998, Lippincott-Raven: Philadelphia, pp. 767–72.

29. Parkes, C., P. Laungani, et al. *Death and Bereavement across Cultures.* 1997, Routledge: New York.

30. Parkes, C., B. Benjamin, et al. Broken heart: Statistical study of increased mortality among widowers. BMJ 1969; 5646: 740–3.

31. Prigerson, H. G. et al. Inventory of Complicated Grief: A scale to measure maladaptive symptoms of loss. Psychiatry Res 1995; 59(1–2): 65–79.

32. Rees, W. The bereaved and their hallucinations. In B.E.A. Schoenberg, ed. *Bereavement—Its Psychosocial Aspects.* 1975, Columbia University Press: New York, pp. 66–71.

33. Rando, T., ed. *Treatment of Complicated Mourning.* 1993, Research Press: Champaign, Ill.

34. Blackman, S. *Graceful Exits—How Great Beings Die.* 1997, Weatherhill: New York.

35. Maluso-Bolton, T. Terminal agitation. Journal of Hospice and Palliative Nursing 2000; 2: 9–19.

36. Lawlor, P.G., R.L. Fainsinger, et al. Delirium at the end of life: Critical issues in clinical practice and research. JAMA 2000; 284(19): 2427–9.

37. Massie, M., J. Holland, et al. Delirium in terminally ill cancer patients. Am J Psychiatry 1983; 140: 1048–50.

38. Enck, R. *The Medical Care of Terminally Ill Patients.* 1994, Johns Hopkins University Press: Baltimore, pp. 32–6.

39. Callahan, M. and P. Kelley. *Final Gifts—Understanding the Special Awareness, Needs and Communications of the Dying.* 1992, Poseidon: New York.

40. McKeith, I. et al. Consensus guidelines for the clinical and pathologic diagnosis of dementia with Lewy bodies. Neurology 1996: 47: 1113–23.

41. Gagnon, P. et al. Delirium in terminal cancer: A prospective study using daily screening, early diagnosis and continuous monitoring. J Pain Symptom Manage 2000; 19(6): 412–26.

42. Grassi, L. et al. Assessing delirium in cancer patients. The Italian versions of the delirium rating scale and the memorial delirium assessment scale. J Pain Symptom Manage 2001: 21(1): 59–68.

43. Lawlor, P. and B. Gagnon. Occurrence, causes, and outcomes of delirium in patients with advanced cancer: A prospective study. Arch Intern Med 2000; 160: 786–94.

44. Breitbart, W. et al. A double-blind trial of haloperidol, chlorpromazine, and lorazepam in the treatment of delirium in hospitalized AIDS patients. Am J Psychiatry 1996; 153(2): 231–7.

45. Breitbart, W. and D. Strout. Delirium in the terminally ill. Clin Geriatr Med 2000; 16(2): 357–72.

46. Quill, T. E. and I. R. Byock. Responding to intractable terminal suffering: The role of terminal sedation and voluntary refusal of food and fluids. ACP-ASIM End-of-Life Care Consensus Panel. American College of Physicians—American Society of Internal Medicine. Ann Intern Med 2000; 132(5): 408–14.

47. Hallenbeck, J. Terminal Sedation—Ethical implications in different situations. Journal of Palliative Medicine 2000; 2: 313–20.

48. Abrahm, J. A *Physician's Guide to Pain and Symptom Management in Cancer Patients*. 2000, Johns Hopkins University Press: Baltimore, pp. 352–4.
49. Weissman, D. E. Fast Fact and Concept #01: Treating terminal delirium. End of LIfe Education Project. http://www.eperc.mcw.edu/, 1999.
50. Wink, P. Addressing end-of-life issues: Spirituality and inner life. GENERATIONS/ Care at the End of Life: Restoring a balance. 1999(Spring): 75–80.
51. Dein, S. and J. Stygall. Does being religious help or hinder coping with chronic illness? A critical literature review. Palliat Med 1997; 11(4): 291–8.
52. King, D. E. and B. Bushwick. Beliefs and attitudes of hospital inpatients about faith healing and prayer. J Fam Pract 1994; 39(4): 349–52.
53. Dowling Singh, K. *The Grace in Dying*. 2000, Harper: San Francisco.
54. Ambuel, B. and D. E. Weissman. Fast Fact and Concept #19: Taking a spiritual history. End of Life Education Project. http://www.eperc.mcw.edu/, 1999.
55. Pulchalski, C. and D. B. Larson. Developing curricula in spirituality and medicine. Acad Med 1998; 73: 970–4.
56. Pulchalski, C. and A. Romer. Taking a spiritual history allows clinicians to understand patients more fully. Journal of Palliative Medicine 2000; 3: 129–37.
57. Baines, B. Relief of suffering at the end of life: looking beyond pain. American Academy of Hospice and Palliative Medicine National Convention. June 29, 2000, Atlanta, Ga.
58. Neuberger, J. Cultural issues in palliative care. In: D. Doyle, G. Hanks, et al. *The Oxford Textbook of Palliative Medicine*. 1998, Oxford University Press: New York, pp. 777–86.
59. Byock, I. R. *Dying Well*. 1997, Riverhead: New York.
60. Steinhauser, K. E. et al. Factors considered important at the end of life by patients, family, physicians, and other care providers. JAMA 2000; 284(19): 2476–82.
61. Steinhauser, K. E. et al. In search of a good death: Observations of patients, families, and providers. Ann Intern Med 2000; 132(10): 825–32.
62. Steinhauser, K. et al. Preparing for the end of life: Preferences of patients, families, physicians, and other care providers. J Pain Symptom Manage 2001; 22(3): 727–37.

8

Communication

The single biggest problem in communication is the illusion that it has taken place.

George Bernard Shaw

We all communicate. We cannot help it. Whenever we are in contact with other people, we send and receive messages. Because we all can communicate, we take communication for granted. We tend to assume that our natural abilities are sufficient. In palliative care this often is not the case; good intentions and personal experience are usually inadequate to rise to the great challenges inherit in this work. Especially at the end of life, the stakes are high. Agonizing decisions must be made. Misunderstandings can easily occur. We encounter taboos and assumptions that obscure communication and comprehension. Communication is dangerous, emotionally charged, and absolutely critical to good palliative care. Advising clinicians to start this drug or that is fairly easy. Working with clinicians, patients, and their families to enhance understanding and facilitate collaborative problem solving through communication is difficult and requires greater skill than does practically anything else we do.

The evidence is overwhelming that clinicians have difficulty communicating well with patients and families in general.[1] For example, Beckman and Frankel analyzed 74 audiotapes of physicians in a general medical clinic talking with patients and found that in only 23% of cases did physicians give patients a chance to fully describe their concerns. On average, patients were interrupted 18 seconds after beginning to talk.[2] In a similar study Waitzkin found that in clinical encounters that lasted on average 16.5 minutes, patients spent an average of 8 seconds asking questions of their physicians. Although physicians believed they spent on average 9 minutes providing information to patients, in fact, they spent less than 40 seconds.[3] This data is striking in the presence of evidence that "information seeking is a foremost goal of patients in primary care."[1,4]

Recently, palliative care literature similarly has documented poor communication by clinicians.[5-8] For example, Tulsky, in reviewing audiotapes of resident physicians discussing resuscitation statuses with patients, found that they often did not relay critical information that was needed for decision making, such as what resuscitation entailed or the probability of successful resuscitation. Even so, physicians dominated the average 10 minutes of speaking time. In only 10% of cases were patient values or goals discussed.[5] Fortunately, studies have also demonstrated that good (or at least better) communication is possible. Roter and colleagues compared audiotaped physician–patient discussions that involved 18 purported expert physicians (as evidenced by publications in bioethics or communication) with 56 academic general internists. As measured by a communication rating scale, the experts were significantly better than were the nonexperts. They were less dominant in conversations, were more likely to engage in partnership building, and paid more attention to psychosocial and lifestyle concerns of patients.[9] Although these studies all relate to physicians, I suspect other health care disciplines share difficulties in communication. It makes sense that if we have trouble communicating effectively even in routine office visits, it will be much more difficult to communicate about the critical issues that routinely arise in the provision of palliative care.

The importance of good communication in palliative care has not been lost on the leaders of palliative care education. Numerous calls have been made for better training in this area.[10-15] The good news is that major educational initiatives to improve the quality of palliative care, such as EPEC (Educating Physicians about End-of-Life Care), End of Life Nursing Education Consortium (ELNEC), Improving Residency Training in End-of-Life Care directed by Dr. David Weissman, faculty development programs in end-of-life care at Harvard, the Program in Palliative Care Education and Practice, and our own End-of-Life (ELC) program at the Stanford Faculty Development Center, devote a great deal of time and effort to improving communication skills.* The bad news is that improving communication skills and demonstrating a lasting

*Websites for education initiatives: EPEC, www.epec.net/; ELNEC, www.aacn.nche.edu/ELNEC/; Improving Residency Training in End of Life Care, www.mcw.edu/pallmed; Stanford Faculty Development Center, http://sfdc.stanford.edu/; Harvard, www.hms.harvard.edu/cdi/pallcare/

effect on clinician behavior is very difficult. Shorr recently published a study that demonstrated no significant difference in the frequency of documentation of end-of-life care issues following an administrative and educational effort to improve both the quality of discussions and their documentation.[16] Although of limited scope and focused on documentation rather than qualitative aspects of communication, this report serves as a warning to those who think that clinicians will necessarily change their ways following brief educational interventions aimed at skill training.

Skill training in communication is important, and certain core skills will be reviewed later in this chapter. However, it is not enough simply to learn how to do something, such as share bad news, as we might learn a technical skill such as catheter insertion. Communication involves dynamic interactions among individuals. We clinicians are not entirely in charge of what happens. How participants understand and view the world and their communication styles will have a profound effect on any given interaction. As Shaw suggested in the epigraph to this chapter, understandings of communication may differ so much that any perception that communication has occurred may be an illusion. Thus, if we are to improve our abilities to communicate with patients and families, who may have very different communication styles from us, we need first to reflect on our own communication styles.

Clinicians are at least "bi-cultural" in communication styles. That is, we learn from childhood certain ways of communicating that are shaped largely by our cultural experience—a blend of ethnicity, national origin, generation, and sex, among other things. In becoming clinicians we are "acculturated" into a new "subculture" of medicine, with its own peculiar communication styles. We learn to pay attention to some things and to ignore others.[17] For example, in learning how to "take a medical history," we learn to ask certain questions to the exclusion of others. We learn to take a *"social* history" that stresses documentation of risky lifestyle behaviors, such as smoking, drinking, and sex, over understanding the patient's social network. We do not even have a *personal* history section in the history and physical to reflect how that patient understands his or her illness or how that patient might characterize himself or herself as a person, helpful though such information might be. In learning how to do a history and physical that stresses the importance of objective data, we also quietly learn that what the patient thinks of his or her condition is largely irrelevant.

In learning medical communication skills such as history taking, we are learning to create certain types of stories relative to episodes of illness. Medical stories tend to favor the objective over the subjective. Logic is valued over emotion. In contrast, patients and families commonly work along very different story lines. As suggested throughout this book, problems tend to arise and miscommunication tends to occur when story lines are grossly out of sync, often to the extent that we end up talking past each other.

The stories we create shape our communication, but they also may have profound effects on what actually happens to people. In particular, our medical stories shape what we do to patients. The power of clinicians' stories was not lost on Anatole Broyard when he contemplated the stories of his physicians in relation to his own story as a patient.

> When a doctor makes a difficult diagnosis, it is not only his medical knowledge that determines it but a voice in his head. Such a diagnosis depends as much on inspiration as art does. Whether he wants to be or not, the doctor is a storyteller, and he can turn our lives into good or bad stories, regardless of the diagnosis. If my doctor would allow me, I would be glad to help him here, to take him on as *my* patient.[18]

In suggesting that he could help the physician by taking him on as his patient, Broyard points to the possibility of collaborative story *writing* (as well as, perhaps, enjoying a reversal in roles in terms of power). If clinicians are to learn to communicate better with their patients and families, they must learn how better to bring into sync the often very different story lines of themselves, patient, and families.

Perhaps this point can be made clearer through a story. Recently, I was asked to do a palliative care consult on an 80-year-old man in an intensive care unit (ICU). The story I first heard, from the resident physician, was that the patient had *presented** to the hospital for an *elective* colonoscopy but was so weak that he began to experience *respiratory failure* and was *emergently intubated*. Subsequent *work-up* revealed that he had advanced metastatic *cancer of unknown primary* (which *carries a grim prognosis*). The ICU team was pessimistic about their ability to *wean* the patient from the ventilator. Remarkably, the patient appeared otherwise comfortable and was reasonably clear thinking, although intubation was a barrier to communication. The team informed him of his grim prognosis and recommended a transition to *comfort care*. When the patient wrote that he wanted *everything done*, the team was in a quandary. The patient's situation was perceived as being *medically futile*, but either the patient did not comprehend this or he had some belief system that required everything to be done. He lacked a *designated surrogate decision maker*, which worried the team because they did not want to be trapped into providing care they believed to be *futile* or even harmful based on this *directive* if or when the patient lost *decision-making capacity*. An ethics consult was obtained, which concurred that the patient seemed to have decision-making capacity and thus that everything should be done for now. The consult team also laid out the rules to follow in that institution for *surrogate decision making*, according to the principle of *sub-*

---

*In this story I italicize some words peculiar to medical storytelling. In this context their use is entirely normal. However, if extracted from this medical context, as they might be if shared with patients and families, their usage seems very odd.

stituted judgment, if or when the patient lost *capacity*. It was at this time that a palliative care consult was ordered. This story was elicited from clinicians, and additional worries were identified, largely concerning procedural questions—"should we put in a feeding tube, should he receive a tracheostomy?"

A fellow on our service had spoken briefly with the patient before I met him and was astute enough to ask what the patient wanted. The patient wrote "Time." He wanted a year to live. When I met Mr. C, he appeared tired and had a small wash towel on his forehead. "Are you comfortable?" I asked. He nodded. My major task in performing this consult was to identify the varying stories among clinicians and the patient and to see to what extent I could bring these stories together into a (hopefully) mutually agreeable story line, so I tried to understand his story. First, I needed to build a relationship whereupon he would be trusting enough to share his story. Storytelling requires a listener, and for very important, personal stories one has to be worthy of hearing. "I heard you are writing a book about China," I said. Again, he nodded. Mr. C shared some of the specifics, and I told him I had been to China and that indeed a book about the subject would be very interesting. I then inquired as to his understanding of his situation. Usually, at this point I will ask an open-ended question such as "What's your understanding of what has happened to you?" However, because of his intubation, I had to rephrase my questions to the extent possible to facilitate yes–no responses. "Did the doctors tell you what is wrong with you?" Nod. "Did they tell you that you have cancer?" Nod. "That must have been hard news, I'm sorry." Double nod, eyes held half-closed for a second. He clearly understood that he had cancer and that it was bad. "Did they say how much time they thought you had left?" Shrug, indicating he was not sure. Our conversation went on like this. Amidst nods, head shakes, shrugs, and brief, written phrases on a scrap of paper, his story was beginning to take form. Clearly, at that time he was still dealing with his dying as if it were a *choice*. When he expressed his wish to live for a year to finish his book, I first validated the wish: "Wouldn't that be great!" I said, and I meant it. I then shared with him the bad news, much along the lines outlined later in the text. "I'm afraid I have some bad news. I do not believe, nor do any of the other doctors, that we have the means to keep you alive for a year. I wish we did. I think you probably have days to, at best, a few weeks to live. Sadly, none of us have the power or medical technology to change that." Mr. C closed his eyes briefly but did not look shocked at what I said. After a pause, I asked, "Are you surprised by what I just said?" He shook his head slowly. If he had been able to communicate more freely, I probably would have asked what was going through his mind. However, his intubation prohibited such an open-ended question. Instead, I tried to imagine myself in his position—what it must have been like to come in for an elective procedure and then wake up in an ICU with a tube in your throat and lots of people in white coats zooming about the place. In trying to empathize (and confirm if this was the way he was experiencing things) I said, "I bet this must all be happening very fast for you." He nodded vigorously, and I sensed more emotion in this response than to the bad news I had given him. "I bet you could just use some time to let this sink in." Again, he nodded.

Palliative Care Note

When patients or families express what you believe to be an unrealistic goal or hope, first validate the wish with a statement such as "Wouldn't that be nice!" Later, you can offer your opinion as to how likely it is that the goal will be obtained.

Time was a major theme in both the ICU team's and the patient's stories. The ICU team saw time, a precious resource, as being wasted in providing futile care. The team was also worried that in time Mr. C would lose decision-making capacity, which would only complicate matters. For Mr. C, time was also running out. However, whatever time was left was seen as a precious resource. I saw an opportunity to bring these stories into sync. I suggested to him that time did indeed appear to be short but that being intubated might keep him alive long enough to accomplish some other tasks, if he had any. He wrote, "What about my estate?" He drew a box with the word *steel* next to it. Misinterpreting, I asked, "Is that a coffin?" He shook his head no. Finally, we figured out he had a steel box at home with his will in it, which he wanted to update. I suggested that we might help get the box. At no time in this conversation did I pressure him to change his mind about the aggressiveness of his care.

I communicated with the ICU team about our conversation and the box. They recognized the shift in goals as a major step forward and launched an effort to retrieve the box. Finally, there was something they could do, and his care was no longer "futile." Their frustration receded. On my next visit Mr. C was visibly glad to see me and happy that efforts were under way to get the box. However, the ICU team was concerned that he was not improving. His sodium level was falling, and it was feared that he might soon lose decision-making capacity. It became clear in our conversations that Mr C's desire to have everything done arose both from concrete goals that had shifted (from a book to revising a will) and his need to have a bit more time to come to grips with what had happened to him. Recognizing this, I first confirmed that, for the time being, he still preferred aggressive life support. He nodded yes. I then asked if we had his permission to shift the focus of his care to comfort from life prolongation *only if* he were "to become unable to meaningfully interact with his environment, and reversal of this state was thought unlikely," as I documented in the chart. Of course, I did not use these words with him. I said something like, "If you get to the point where you are seriously ill and dying and have no idea what is going on, and if it looks like the docs can't get you back to your current condition, do we have your permission to switch gears from working to prolong your life to exclusively focusing on your comfort with no effort to prolong your life? This would include stopping life support." He clearly nodded yes. Because of the communication barrier caused by his intubation, I asked the question in other ways and confirmed his understanding of what I had proposed. This conversation was witnessed. This "advance, advance directive" (on top of his current advance directive for maximal support) describing a not-unlikely scenario, made sense in that his desire to continue life support was linked to explicit goals that he wanted to accomplish. If he were to become unable to accomplish such goals, then there would be little point to continue life support. When this conversation (and possible story line) was conveyed to the ICU, they were much relieved, as this addressed an issue of tension in their story line.

The box was found, and Mr. C got some time to come to grips. It looked as if he might be "weanable" from the ventilator, but the ICU team felt they needed to understand before extubation whether they should reintubate him if medically required following extubation. As their story lines came together, the ICU team was able to discuss this with Mr. C, and after a few days he consented to extubation without reintubation and a transition to comfort care only. He was successfully extubated and moved to hospice, where he died peacefully two days later.

In reading the following descriptions of communication skills, the reader is advised to keep in mind that such discrete skills will be most effective if they are employed within a much larger context of human relations and storytelling. And, as with any skill, they require practice, practice, practice.

ABCs of Communication

Stepping back from issues of storytelling, I now return to basics. Why do we communicate? At a simple level we share data. Even for communication as simple as data transfer, there must be a connection between those who wish to communicate with each other. This connection, like a computer modem, may be strong and reliable or weak, with a fuzzy signal that occasionally goes down. Both sender and receiver must agree to certain standards of language for successful transfer. Even this will not guarantee that a message, successfully transmitted, will actually be understood. Understanding requires an ability to get beyond the data to meaning, which may or may not be shared between sender and receiver, and this is the simple part! For human beings communication is considerably more complicated. Communication involves *relationships* and *contexts*. We are not mindless terminals linked by cables. A certain glance can represent a threat or a come-on. We often communicate in order to get our way or to dominate a relationship. Communication can be about power. We may be less interested in the other person understanding our position than in his or her acquiescing to it. At times we reach out to each other for companionship and solace. Sometimes we talk just to talk. While a computer cable exists only for the transmission of electronic signals, humans use the means of communication and the "box" within which communication occurs as part of the message. Our choice, whether to call on the telephone, send an e-mail, speak in a hallway, or sequester ourselves in a family conference is not just a means of communication, it is part of the message.

Some observations about communication between clinicians (especially doctors) and patients and their families are:

- Physicians (and other clinicians) talk too much and do not listen enough.
- Physicians tend to focus exclusively on the cognitive (thinking) aspects of communication and ignore affective (emotional) aspects.[19]
- Physicians tend to force their agendas over patient and family agendas.

Dealing with Emotions and Empathy

As outlined above, physicians tend to be most comfortable addressing cognitive aspects of communication. Dealing with the emotions that arise in others and in oneself is considerably more difficult. Why is this so? Some emotions are simply hard to deal with for practically anyone—anger and sorrow, for example. Clinicians face an additional barrier, or handicap. Doctors (as well as nurses, social workers, and others) are professionals, and with this professional role comes a lot of baggage. We are scientists. We are in charge, and we are rational. To a degree, this is all true, but we are also human. Our humanity may be viewed by some as a weakness, a failing in our professional role. However, this humanity is central to the relational aspect of communication with our patients and their families. In a crisis patients and families *want* the professional. They want clear thinking, and they want our professional skills. They also want a human being with whom they can relate.

Patients and families often try to talk our language. They try to speak "doctor-talk" requesting an IV when the subtext is really "I'm feeling desperate, please help me!" They, too, may be more comfortable dealing with the cognitive aspects of communication and may avoid emotional issues. Choosing when to address the emotional subtext is an art; there are times to do it and times not to do so. It is safe to say that most physicians do not do it enough and lack the skills to know how to address the emotional subtext.

Techniques for dealing with and exploring emotions

Naming or mirroring. One way of addressing emotions in another is simply to name what you see or think you see: "You seem very angry." Here, you are inviting the other person to raise what has been a subtext to the text.

Identifying the mood. In hearing a sad story, one might reflect "How sad." Such a statement reflects a feeling shared by speaker and listener as well as the mood in the room and in this subtle way differs from naming. It is also an empathetic response (see below on empathy). Identifying the mood draws attention to a common emotional context and the relationships among participants as an aspect of communication.

Further exploration. Addressing affect does not mean just bringing it out in the open; it is not simple catharsis. Affect can be explored cognitively. One can expand the conversation by inviting further exploration of an emotion: "Where do you think your sadness is coming from?" or "What is it that makes you so angry?" An empathetic statement is also an effective way to invite exploration: "It must be really hard to see your dad like this."

Sharing our own emotions. Now we're on scary ground. "Getting emotional" suggests a loss of control that threatens our professional roles, and we will be considered poor clinicians if we routinely "lose it" with our patients. How can we authentically share our emotions and yet be true to the maxim that in the clinician–patient relationship, the needs of the patient (and family) come first? We must acknowledge that, as human beings, we will sometimes lose it. It cannot be helped. If a doctor told me he or she had never "lost-it," I would worry about that doctor.[20] Either that doctor is a saint or has built such thick calluses around his or her emotions that I would wonder if accessing those emotions were even possible. Saints are in short supply, so we should consider sharing our emotions from a therapeutic perspective: how could sharing our emotions be helpful to the patient (and family)?

If the emotional subtext of a conversation is completely ignored or suppressed, the situation becomes increasingly unreal and dishonest. This can have a very negative effect. At a time when patients and families are struggling with their emotions, we should not serve as models by running away from ours. Difficult as such emotions can be, bringing them out in the open in a manner that still demonstrates professionalism can simply acknowledge a tension between the doctor and the other that must be dealt with if a relationship is to exist and flourish. It is possible to model being angry, for example, without "losing" it and at the same time express a desire to be helpful: "I'm angry at you because you often demand this or that. It is hard for me to help you when I always feel on the defensive."

What about sharing other emotions, such as grief? We may think behaviors such as crying are undignified. Although people from different cultures likely have different values about this, consider how you might feel if a physician shed a few tears when pronouncing a loved one of yours. Would you consider it unprofessional or a tribute?

Empathy

Technically, empathy refers to an intimate connection with another person such that one experiences the other's emotions as one's own. In seeing someone cry, we cry. In seeing someone in pain, we experience pain. I will leave it to philosophers to argue whether we really can experience someone else's suffering. What is clear is that we can find a certain *resonance* with the emotional states of others. When we respond to a person empathetically, we display verbally and nonverbally this resonance—or at the very least our effort to resonate with that person's experience. Most difficult discussions in palliative and end-of-life care offer numerous opportunities for empathetic responses.[19] Empathetic responses address the affective aspect of communication but go beyond naming or sharing one's own emotions, as discussed above. The emphasis is on resonance. Many empathetic responses require no words, being best communicated nonverbally. For example, our voices may choke up. We may stand silently by a grieving widow as she sobs by the bedside of her now deceased husband. We may use physical touch, such as holding a hand just a second longer than is customary. Occasionally we may hug, although judgment must be used as to who is a "hugger" and who is not. Even how we cover a patient after an examination may display empathy or lack thereof. Listening, we stay in contact with the other. When pain or sorrow arises, we may change position or furrow a brow. Verbally, we may express at least an effort to understand the hardship of the other. To the family member keeping vigil, one might say, "You must be exhausted. Did you sleep last night?" When a relative comes from far away and seems surprised at how a loved one has changed, "How long has it been since you've seen your father? This must come as quite a shock." A more directly empathetic statement (but not necessarily better) might more overtly reflect your resonance with the other's state: "I really feel for you. I share your sadness," or simply, "How sad." One last piece of advice—if you do offer an empathetic response, makes sure it is genuine. False empathy is worse than no empathy at all.

Agendas

Communication is controlled, consciously or unconsciously, by participants, who signal where they wish to go. Like choosing a fork in the road, one can choose to turn left or right. The other participant can choose to follow or ignore this lead. Being conscious of these choices and the other's response enhances communication. Choosing to address cognitive rather than affective content in an exchange is an example of such a choice. Another choice is whether to expand a certain conversational thread or to terminate it. A phrase suggesting expansion might be "Tell me more about that." Silence itself may suggest the opportunity for expansion or may be used to signal the end of a conversation thread. A terminating or finishing phrase might be "Let's talk more about that tomorrow" or "Yes, but let's get back to what we were talking about," to suggest a return to an earlier conversational thread. Standing up and offering one's hand suggests a termination as well. Skill is required to know when to expand a discussion, when to end it, and how.

Agendas arise to a large degree from a person's story line. We all attempt to "follow the plot" of a story of our own construction. If participants in a conversation have radically different story lines with different plots moving toward different endings, the tendency is to "force" the other along one's own story line. A physician following a story line of "doing an history and physical," for example, might impose this particular story line on a patient and family who may be working from very different story lines that may range from the complex ("I need to understand why this happened to me") to the most practical ("I need to go to the bathroom"). It is quite remarkable the extent to which patients and families will cooperate with such impositions. When the other does not cooperate with one's agenda, the choices are limited—to be more forceful (loud, angry speech, threatening, etc.), to cut off attempts at communication, or, as seems particularly common in clinical settings, to continue talking as if communication were happening when, in fact, people are talking past one another and, perpetuating the illusion of communication, as Shaw put it. To the extent that story lines are to come into sync, this process must entail an ability to recognize one's own agenda and an ability to suspend this agenda, at least temporarily, while attending to the agenda of the other. I now consider some of the more specific communication issues and skills in palliative care.

Sharing Bad News

One of the most difficult tasks a clinician faces is the sharing of bad news: "Mr. Jones, I've some bad news; the biopsy came back positive for cancer." On call in the middle of the night, you rush to a code. Despite all efforts, the patient dies. Your job is to call the patient's husband or wife, mother or father. Even moments of great joy may contain the seeds of immense sorrow: "Mrs. Smith, I'm sorry, there is something wrong with the baby. . . ."

Few would deny the importance of sharing such news, yet historically very little training has been offered to clinicians to help them improve their ability to give bad news. Rarely is it included in formal course work in the preclinical years of medical school. One could reasonably argue that such training should occur during clinical training. However, there is evidence that sharing bad news is rarely modeled by attending physicians, who, in theory, have had the most experience with this task. For example, in a recent survey we conducted of medical interns,

5 of 27 (19%) interns surveyed reported *never* having seen an attending physician share bad news, 4 of 27 (15%) reported seeing it once, 12 of 27 (44%) reported seeing this two to three times, and only 6 of 27 (22%) reported seeing this four or more times.[21] Similar findings exist in the literature for other disciplines, such as surgery.[22] Given the frequency with which bad news must be shared, these rates are remarkably low. Informal discussions with house staff suggest that physicians-in-training learn on their own or from other physicians-in-training. Learning to give bad news has become part of the hidden curriculum for residents in training, part of the resident subculture.[23] This is clearly far from ideal. Teachers in the field largely agree that certain steps should be followed in sharing bad news with minor variations.[24-29]

Preparation

1. To the greatest extent possible, bad news should be shared in person. Sometimes we have no choice but to share bad news by telephone. However, if possible, sharing in person is far preferable. Cryptic and scary urgent calls such as, "Mrs. Jones, you must come in right away, I've got to talk with you," should be avoided if at all possible. When doing a lab test or procedure with a high probability that bad news will result, one might schedule a follow-up meeting that will quickly follow test availability. Or one might advise a patient or family that regardless of good or bad news, they will be called to come in to discuss the results. It is usually advisable to have a support person there for the person receiving bad news, if possible.

2. Find a quiet place, minimize distractions, and allow adequate time. It can be incredibly difficult to find a quiet place without distractions. Often, one must improvise. Try to find a chair for yourself and the other person(s). Sitting down shows you are paying attention and not about to rush somewhere else. Avoid speaking in hallways and while on the run. Notify staff that you do not wish to be interrupted. Set your beeper on vibration mode. Be honest about how much time it will take to address the bad news, and set that time aside. A quiet setting, often in stark contrast with the usual noisy, hectic world of medicine, also establishes a context that is respectful but communicates that something important is about to happen.

3. Do your homework. Have needed medical information available. If unfamiliar with the implications of the bad news, find out what you can. Identify special issues or barriers that might interfere with communication—language or cognitive disorders, for example—and attempt to compensate (have a translator available if a language barrier exists). If referral is needed and follow-up appointments need to be scheduled, have these planned to the extent possible before sharing bad news.

Making a Connection

Especially if the person to receive bad news suspects or believes bad news is coming, do not drag out introductions. However, you do need to make a connection with the person. Certain tasks that frequently come up in this important but usually brief stage are:

1. Introductions. Introduce yourself and any others with you. If others are present who you do not know, find out who they are.
2. Assess the recipient's status. Inquire about his or her comfort and immediate needs. As in other communication, you may wish to assess the recipient's understanding of the situation. This will not only help you make the transition to sharing the news but will help you assess the patient's perception of the circumstances. You might start with, "What is your understanding of what has happened" (or why a test was done, etc.)? Buckman has suggested that we assess what the recipient is willing and able to hear.[26]

Sharing the News

Really bad news is like a neutron bomb. The "radiation" produced allows only the simplest messages to penetrate all the static.

1. Speak slowly. Use clear, unambiguous language.
2. Give an advance alert. You might say, "I'm afraid I have some bad news. . . ." Pause only a couple of seconds after this.
3. Give the news. This should be very brief at this stage, only a few short sentences: "The biopsy didn't turn out as we had hoped. It revealed cancer."

The Aftermath

1. Await the reaction quietly. Be prepared for the unexpected. Recipients may respond in a variety of unpredictable ways. They may cry, faint, scream, be silent, laugh, or immediately ask factual questions. They may even appear not to have heard you. Whatever the response, let it happen. Be present and connect. Do *not* try to compensate for your own discomfort by talking to fill this most uncomfortable space.
2. Watch and listen for a signal that they want you to respond. The signal may be a question or a sign that they are open to an empathetic response. Responses should remain fairly simple at this stage. Respect the shock. Avoid the temptation to monopolize the encounter with a lot of data, such as all the possible therapeutic options. Sometimes physicians will try to *use* the shock to unburden additional bad news or details. They may think, "Might as well get it over with and tell it all," or they may think that pro-

viding details will compensate somehow for the shock and engender hope. You may assess the person's reaction with a direct inquiry: "This must be hard for you. What is going through your mind now?"

3. Follow the person's lead. Some recipients can handle more new information than can others. Generally, you should validate the person's reaction. Bad news usually means that the person's world has just been turned upside down. The sudden loss of any semblance of control is part of this initial shock. You may help reestablish some control by following the person's lead: "Would you like more information now or should we talk later?" "Who would you like to come be with you?" This need to reestablish some control must be balanced against the reality that many recipients are very fragile and will need help even with very basic things. You can inquire how you could best be of help: "Is there someone we can call for you?"

Transition to Follow-Up

1. Schedule a follow-up meeting. Have a concrete plan for follow-up in the very near future (often later that day or within a couple of days—*not* a month later). This follow-up meeting is a good time to address more specific questions that will arise and to share more detailed information. The recipient may be given tasks to accomplish before the meeting. You may ask if they wish a support person to be present (if not already involved) or that they write down concerns or questions: "Why don't you write down any questions you have for that meeting."

2. Be clear about what your role will be in the process and who will be available for support. If you are going to be in it for the duration (perhaps as a primary caregiver for a newly diagnosed terminal illness), tell the patient that you will be there for him or her. If you are going to hand off support to another, be clear about who that person will be and how contact will be made. Clarify what the relationships will be among the patient, the new caregiver, and youself. Help facilitate this new connection.

3. As you began, so should you end. As the encounter draws to a close, look for a way to leave with an empathetic connection. Let the recipient know you care.

Pay Attention To and Respect Your Own Feelings and Needs

I purposely used the term *sharing* bad news rather than *giving* to highlight that we share in the pain that comes with bad news.[30] To the extent we empathize with the receiver of the news, we will hurt. We also have our own physician and clinician pains. We like to be able to fix things and tend to be perfectionists. Facing bad news means acknowledging that we cannot fix everything. If the patient's earlier health care was less than perfect, which it may have been, or if mistakes were made, as occasionally happens, we feel terrible. At the very least, sharing bad news (and doing it well) requires huge amounts of energy and may leave us feeling drained.

Our profession leaves little time or space to attend to our own needs and feelings. However, we ignore them at our peril. I have no simple recipe for *how* to attend to such needs any more than I can suggest where to find a chair to sit with your patient. You may take a few minutes' time out and walk in the garden. You may go to your call room and cry or take a shower. Perhaps you will pray or meditate. I have found that finding a friend or colleague with whom to talk is very valuable. Most clinicians I know are far harder on themselves than on anyone else. Usually, support is best offered by another in the same profession. Some of the anguish in a profession can only be understood by another in the same profession. When in doubt, be kind to yourself.

For all the pain associated with sharing bad news, such news draws us back to our common humanity. In such situations being a doctor or a nurse is not enough. The issues raised by bad news exist for all of us. We all will receive bad news. We all will suffer loss and eventually die. I suspect it is this truth that we most fear. It is understandable that we might want to run away. However, to the extent we can engage our hearts in the process of sharing bad news, with all the hopes and fears this entails, we will, I believe, become better clinicians and better people.

Incorporating Patient and Family Preferences into Difficult Decisions

Making difficult decisions is part of the work of medicine. Good decision making depends on a variety of factors, including knowledge and clinical reasoning skills. Deciding which antibiotic to use or what particular surgical approach to follow are examples of difficult decisions that require professional expertise on the part of the clinician. In caring for very sick and dying patients, decisions are particularly difficult because professional expertise and opinion mix with very personal *choices* on the part of patients and families. Whether a feeding tube should be placed is not just a technical problem or a dispassionate weighing of known benefits, burdens, and probabilities.[31] Patient and family preferences must be incorporated into the process if a good decision is to be made.

Mr. C, who was introduced at the beginning of this chapter, and the ICU staff faced such a difficult decision—should aggressive life support be continued or not. This decision was not a purely medical decision but revolved around Mr. C's understanding of his condition and his goals for the future. Clinicians encounter many such decisions that require patient and family participation. What is the patient's resuscitation status, full code or DNR? Should a further round of chemotherapy be tried? Should a patient with chronic obstructive pulmonary disease and recurrent admissions to the ICU be electively intubated during the next medical decompensation? Should a feeding tube be placed in a patient who has swallowing difficulties? Should a patient be referred to hospice? Should a patient be transferred from the nursing home to the acute hospital? Should antibiotics or IVs be used if a patient develops pneumonia? Studies suggest that physicians do a poor job when talking with patients about relatively straightforward medical decisions.[32] How much more difficult these decisions must be!

Difficult decisions can be understood to represent major branches in patients' story lines. Depending on which road is taken, the patient's life will change in profound ways. For example, being admitted to home hospice has multiple effects on the system of care for the patient and family. Beyond this, the symbolism involved in being admitted to hospice may allow patients and families to acknowledge that dying is actually happening and result in dramatic changes in how they deal with the illness and one another.

Many physicians are extremely ambivalent about incorporating patient and family preferences into difficult decisions. Some years ago I was teaching a mixed group of physicians and nonphysicians about how to discuss patients' resuscitation statuses. I asked everybody, "Do you think we should incorporate patient preferences into these decisions?" All nodded in the affirmative. I then addressed only the physicians: "Physicians. Be honest. *When* do you ask a patient about their preferences? Do you ask all seriously ill people or only those who *you* think should have a DNR status?" They sheepishly admitted it was usually when they thought a DNR order was a good idea. The lay members were appalled to hear this. Before we collectively lambaste the medical profession on this point, perhaps we should consider more deeply this ambivalence.

Most physicians tend to agree, in principle, about patients' rights to be involved in decision making. However, many also are skeptical of the lay public's ability to make intelligent decisions about health care. Some would say that proper incorporation of preferences means that the physician suggest a therapy and the patient agree, a process called informed consent.

Informed consent, as it is commonly understood, is a process whereby the physician suggests a therapy or procedure and the patient (or proxy) consents. Many clinicians have taken a very literal interpretation of informed consent and construe it to be the completion of a form required for certain invasive procedures. A lumbar puncture (the doctor's idea) is consented to by the patient, who signs a form.* Medical culture has required such form signing for certain pro-

---

*It is interesting that a considerably more invasive procedure, cardiopulmonary resuscitation, does not require informed consent, usually on the basis that this is an *emergency* procedure that cannot be anticipated and thus is exempt from standard guidelines that require consent. That this is *not* the case for many seriously ill patients is something with which current policies have not yet come to grips.

cedures but not for others. A less literal interpretation of informed consent would mean that *any* additional therapies or changes in the plan of care would require the understanding and agreement of the patient or proxy. Such an interpretation certainly expands expectations for patient or proxy involvement. However, this interpretation is still a very narrow way of construing an incorporation of preferences. The physician remains the primary decision maker. The patient's job is to *consent* (or not).

There is some wisdom in this approach. Most physicians can tell horror stories of patients and families who have ordered very specific therapies, much like ordering a pizza: "I want antibiotics with a side-order of intravenous fluid to go." This extreme of consumerism is very difficult for physicians, who often think such orders are ludicrous. They (we) resent being treated like short-order cooks. In other fields of medicine this is a minor annoyance. If a patient presented to a surgeon with abdominal pain and insisted on an appendectomy for something clearly not appendicitis, the surgeon would probably feel quite comfortable refusing and say the procedure "is not indicated." In end-of-life care things are more complicated. Many hospital and health care policies *presume* the almost absolute primacy of the patient or proxy regarding end-of-life decisions. Clinicians may feel strongly that intubation, cardiopulmonary resuscitation (CPR), or antibiotics are "not indicated," yet most hospitals (and society) treat these decisions very differently. No matter how strongly "not indicated" CPR might be considered by clinicians, many hospitals see the full code choice as an absolute right of the patient that cannot be abrogated. The message is: decisions at the end of life are somehow different from other medical decisions; patients and their families are in charge. I think most of us would agree this is not such a bad thing, in and of itself. You may think, "That's the way I want it to be for me!" The problem, as doctors are fully aware, is that sometimes patients and families make very, very foolish choices—not that this is a surprise; people make foolish choices everyday. However, physicians and other clinicians may feel *coerced* into providing treatment that they feel is of little, if any, benefit. Indeed, sometimes we feel coerced into doing things we feel will be downright harmful, and that feels really awful.

Hence, physicians are rightly wary of extreme consumerism. If that is what "incorporating preferences" means, they (and I) want nothing to do with it. On the other hand, the narrow "informed consent" approach preferred by many physicians serves equally poorly. If a patient prefers to die at home rather than in the hospital, is this something for the physician to offer (like a procedure) and to which the patient must consent? I think not. The issue for many seriously ill and dying patients is not so much a choice of this procedure or that or whether to take out an appendix or not, but how that person and that family want to live and to die. Patient and family wishes and values are not some peripheral issue, they are the main issue.

Fortunately, in most cases there is a middle ground between these extremes of consumerism and physician paternalism. Most patients and families will willingly enter into a collaborative decision-making process if offered the chance.

The GOOD acronym (goals, options, opinion, document) provides a construct for communicating with patients and others involved in making such difficult decisions. GOOD decision making for such problems is a cooperative venture that involves input from patients, families, and health care providers. The acronym provides only a crude structure for engaging in such conversations. Flexibility and *practice* are required if communication skills are to improve.

The GOOD Acronym: 'Its *Good* to Incorporate Patient and Family Preferences into Decision Making.'

G: Goals

What are the "big picture" goals for patients, families, and care providers? Understanding the big picture is critical to good decision making and facilitates the identification of explicit treatment goals. Often, these goals are not clearly stated by participants and may not even be clearly conceptualized. Identifying and clarifying such goals makes consideration of specific options much easier. Sometimes goals can be obvious. A patient who shows up at an emergency room with a cut on the finger probably wants it sewn up. We can assume this is a goal we share with the patient. Rarely are goals so clear-cut toward the end of life. Patients and their families may have very different goals relating to how they wish to live and die. Often, we are simply unaware of patient and family goals because such goals arise from long and complex life stories about which we are understandably ignorant. We will not understand their goals unless we ask. In terms of storytelling, goals represent possible story endpoints.

Steps in considering goals include:

- Identify stakeholders. Whose goals do you need to consider? The patient's goals are most important, but the goals of others are also relevant. Which family members are involved, and what are their relationships to the patient? Are spiritual or community leaders active participants? What clinicians, physicians, and other health professionals are involved in the patient's care and decision making? Whose stories do you need to consider?
- Elucidate stakeholders' understanding. Stakeholders' goals for the future make sense only relative to *current* understandings. Consider asking a patient (or relative), "What is your understanding of . . ." (your current condition, your illness, why you are here)? A related but distinct question is, "What have you been told about your condition/illness." A patient may have been *told* one thing but have a very different understanding of what is going on. By analogy, imag-

ine getting a phone call from someone asking directions to your place. The goal is clear— to get a certain place. You would first ask, "Where are you now?" If there was some uncertainty as to the person's location, you might ask, "Where do you *think* you are now?" Then and only then could you give intelligent directions depending on his or her location. If there were serious disagreement among fellow travelers as to where they thought they were, it would be impossible to decide on a route no matter how clear the final destination.

Palliative Care Note

"What is your understanding of . . ." is one of the most important questions you can ask regarding an episode of illness.

- Clarify "big picture" goals *first*. A common mistake is to rush too quickly to discussion/argument over specific therapies or options before the big picture is considered. This is like arguing about which highway to take before you have decided where you are going. For example, before discussing the use of antibiotics in a terminally ill patient with a particular infection, it can be very helpful to understand the relative priority of life prolongation compared to a more exclusive focus on comfort without life prolonging efforts. You might say something such as, "I'm trying to understand how you see the big picture. We'll get to the specific decisions we have to address in a moment. Do you have a major goal in your care? What is most important to you?" In considering aggressiveness of life-prolonging interventions, you might ask something such as, "Imagine a line where at one end we would work as hard as we can and aggressively as we can to prolong your life. We would still work to keep you as comfortable as possible, but the priority would be on prolonging your life. At the other end of the line we would work just as hard, focusing on your comfort, but would not attempt to prolong your life at all. In my experience people with your condition might be at either end of this line or anywhere in the middle. Where do you think you are?" For patients unable to conceptualize this spectrum, you might break the line into thirds, saying, "Some people would like everything possible done to prolong life, some people would like modest means used to prolong life, and some would not want their life prolonged at all. To which group do you see yourself belonging?" Big picture goals can be thought of as a final destination along a journey (or story). If one understands what this ultimate destination is, it is much easier to proceed by choosing a general route that may reveal several derivative decisions about where to stop along the way. A note of caution: Do not be surprised if patients and families are confused when you ask them about their goals. This does not necessarily mean that you are communicating poorly. Patients and families are no more used to being asked such questions than clinicians are used to asking them. Indeed, patients and families can become "medicalized" such that they get too caught up in a series of actions, bouncing from one test or procedure to the next, without ever considering what they are trying to accomplish.

- Assess values that guide big picture goals. What is important to the individual? What is desired and what feared? How do these values make sense and guide this person's decision making? Assessing values fleshes out the context within which a specific decision is being made. For example, in the case of Mr. C, understanding the importance to him of finishing his book helped us understand his goal of living for an additional year.

- Identify option-specific goals. Having identified relevant treatments or the options available (see the section on options below), what does the individual hope to accomplish? Is there something in particular that the individual wishes to avoid or fears? Different individuals who consider the same treatment or option will have very different understandings of what will happen if the option is used or not. Similarly, they may have very different hopes and fears relative to the outcomes of particular choices. Although it is important to bear in mind one's ultimate "destination" in a voyage (or story), value in the trip is often found along the way, not just at the very end. This step usually follows the identification of specific options, as discussed below. It is included here for organizational purposes. In real interactions one often must move from considerations of goals to options to values in a more fluid manner. In responding to a request for antibiotics for a patient who is actively dying, for example, if the inquirer's goal of care is the provision comfort only, one can then ask how the person imagines that antibiotics will contribute to comfort.

O: Options

- Start by making a mental list of relevant options to consider. Is there a logical order in which these options should be considered? Although many specific options may emerge, a natural hierarchy usually suggests itself, often from considering big picture goals. A clear decision on one major option will often resolve a subordinate option. If, for example, a decision is made to stop dialysis, yielding a predicted life expectancy of 10 to 14 days, decisions related to many other potential options will then become clearer.

- Inquire if stakeholders are considering options other than those on your list. The ultimate list of options to be considered should be constructed from those of all relevant stakeholders.

- Discuss benefits and burdens. Up until now the focus has been on eliciting the hopes, fears, and opinions of others involved in decisions. Now is the time to offer information about the possible benefits and burdens of taking or not taking an action under consideration. Before doing this it is critical to do your homework. Often clinicians engage in discussions about difficult decisions in this area without knowing basic facts. For example, in discussing a possible DNR status, what is the chance of surviving an attempt at resuscitation? What chance is there of surviving but having significant brain damage? What data exist (or do not exist) relative to tube feeding and the chance of preventing aspiration pneumonia in a patient with abnormal swallowing? What are the pros and cons of treating patients who are actively dying with antibiotics and IV hydration? How would hospice care be different from standard home care? Benefits and burdens only make sense relative to goals. Prolongation of life, for example, may be seen as either a benefit or a burden depending on one's overall goals and values.*

- Consider probability. For many patients understanding the probability of success or failure will be important in deciding on a particular course of action. For example, patients frequently overestimate the overall success rate of CPR and may reconsider their choice for CPR if informed that for patients in similar situations, less than 1% leave the hospital alive following resuscitative efforts. On the other hand, some patients appear to place little value on probability in making medical decisions. Some patients will not care if the chance of successful resuscitation is one in a billion—they will want resuscitative efforts. (Others will decline resuscitation efforts even if guaranteed of success.) It appears that for many patients and families, how a decision and related outcome states fit into their particular stories is as important or more important than are raw probabilities of particular outcome states.[31] For example, a person may base a decision on whether to have resuscitation attempted more on his view of himself as a "fighter" (or not) or his belief that his affairs are in order (or not) than on probability estimates.
- Honor values. Values refer to the relative importance, or weight, that may be attached to particular outcome states. How important is it to be able to live at home? How important is it to be able to eat by mouth (in a patient for whom tube feeding is being considered)? In terms of patient and family stories, again, values provide context and meaning within which characters act and plots unfold. Although the clinician can provide information on potential benefits and burdens of proposed actions, the relative weight of these outcomes arises primarily from the values of the patient and family. If, for example, one of the few residual pleasures left in life is eating, this must be weighed in considering possible tube feeding. Conversely, if the family believes that not providing nutrition when technically possible will be tantamount to starving

---

*Clinicians who would never think about addressing a therapy "outside their area of expertise," such as what chemotherapy agent to use for a particular tumor, often seem not to hesitate to bring up such issues and offer options regarding end-of-life decisions about which they are at least as ignorant. Perhaps this is because they do not recognize that a body of knowledge also exists in this area.

a patient to death, this must be acknowledged and considered. Patient and family values may be particularly misunderstood when patients and clinicians are from different backgrounds. Care must be taken to elicit values in a nonjudgmental way. At the same time, the clinician should consider carefully his or her own values relative to the question at hand. Although some clinicians may like to think that their preferences for certain decisions are based entirely on rational processes and probabilities associated with scientific understanding, this is untrue. We bring to clinical encounters very human values that shape our preferences.

O: Opinion

- Offer your opinion. So far, you have largely listened to others and probably shared some information that may be important in considering specific decisions, such as possible benefits and burdens. Now it is the time to offer your opinion. Although patients and families welcome your involving them, they also usually welcome a clearly stated opinion as to which option(s) might be best.
- Separate data from opinion. Sometimes clinicians pretend to be neutral when, in fact, they have strong beliefs as to what course of action would be best. Certain choices, especially those regarding end-of-life care, have become culturally framed for clinicians in such a way that the issues are seen as entirely personal and outside the boundaries of medicine.° Thinking that it might be improper to offer an opinion in such cases, clinicians may subconsciously avoid sharing data that would lead patients to a desired choice while avoiding stating an opinion directly. This practice is to be discouraged. Consider the two following examples as ways of "shading" data: "If you want us to smash your chest and jam a tube down your throat, hey—that's up to you. Don't let me bias you," or, "We can massage your heart and slip a small breathing tube in to assist your breathing. You want to breathe, don't you? But of course, it is up to you." It would be better to use more neutral language in giving data accompanied by a separate, clear opinion: "Cardiopulmonary resuscitation, or CPR, involves pressing on your chest and inserting a breathing tube. . . ." "In my opinion you would be best served by not having resuscitation attempted (or having it attempted)."
- Explain your opinion, incorporating data from earlier discussions. Try to link your opinion to patient and family views, clinician goals, benefits and burdens of care, probabilities of outcomes, and the values of those involved. You might say something like, "You've told me that quality of life is the most im-

---

°Although the boundary between the personal and the "medical" in such decisions is indeed difficult to demarcate, I do not believe such issues are so outside the medical realm that opinion should not be offered. The choices involve clinicians, and their medical knowledge and experience should help people make more intelligent choices.

portant thing to you. There isn't good evidence that a feeding tube will improve your quality of life. You've told me that eating gives you great pleasure, so in your case, I'd recommend against a feeding tube." In terms of stories, this is your chance to suggest a change in the story line and to bring together divergent story lines. Suggested changes in a story line for patients, families, and clinicians will be accepted only if others understand the change as a reasonable alterative to their own stories. In the case of Mr. C, when I suggested that he might not want continued aggressive life support if he were permanently "out of it," he accepted this, I think, precisely because it made sense in terms of his own story line. His goal for wanting everything done at that time was to revise his will and come to grips with his situation, neither of which would be possible if he were "out of it." My opinion that continued short-term ventilation was not futile was accepted by the ICU team because a concrete, but alternative, goal had been established with which they could help. This was acceptable within their story line.

D: Document

A quick survey of many hospital and clinic charts will reveal that documentation of important discussions is often lacking. This is not only ill advised clinically, but also medically and legally. Imagine a patient with whom you have discussed code status who agrees to a DNR status. She then dies. A relative subsequently states that the patient had always wanted "everything done." The first source of information would be the medical record. A (common) note stating simply "DNR" would not document that the patient had been involved in the decision. You might be sued. Conversely, if you wrote only "Full Code" or nothing at all and the patient arrested and was resuscitated with serious neurologic sequelae, you might be accused of resuscitating a patient against her wishes. The family might refuse to pay the bill. What you should document in your note should include:

- A list of the participants in the discussion and decision.
- A brief account of the essence of the discussion, with attention to the final decision. A note regarding possible tube feeding might say, "I discussed tube feeding with the patient and his daughter. Possible benefits and burdens were identified. I recommended against tube feeding at this time, and patient and daughter agreed."
- If discussing advance care planning, pay attention to both what the patient wants now (a *current* advance directive) as well as what the patient might like if certain things happen (an *advance* advance directive). For example, many patients would like an attempt at resuscitation to be made. However, many, if not most, would like a switch to comfort care if it became clear that the chance of recovery to a reasonable quality of life was very low, as was the case

for Mr. C. You might write something such as, "At this time the patient would like resuscitation attempted. However, he agrees that were he thought to be permanently unable to interact meaningfully with his environment, then he would like only comfort care at that time." A statement such as this can be worth its weight in gold for the patient in the ICU who is not thought likely to recover following resuscitative efforts.

- Make sense of the decision. Was the decision in keeping with an advance directive? Why else does this make sense? This is your chance to write a short story. Such stories can be very brief and state something such as, "This decision makes sense as the patient and family understand he is dying and that their primary goal is now quality of life," or, "This decision is in keeping with the patient's written advance directive."

Communicating with Patients and Families about Hastened Death

Some of the most difficult decisions faced by patients, families, and physicians arise when a request is made to hasten the death of a dying patient. Physician assisted suicide (PAS) is usually considered an ethical controversy.[33,34] Here, I will not discuss the ethics of PAS or attempt to resolve the controversy, but in keeping with the theme of this section, I will offer some suggestions for responding to requests for a hastened death.[35,36]

"Doctor, can you help me get it over with?"
" I'm tired of all this, isn't there something you can give me?"
"Will you help me when my time comes?"
"Hey doc, what about that little black pill?"
"What do you say, how about we get the show on the road?"
"I want to die. Can you give me something?"

Sometimes patients indicate very clearly that they want assistance in hastening their deaths. More often, in my experience, patients toss out very subtle hints that they would like to discuss the issue. Patients may say simply, "I'm tired of all this," or "I wonder how long this dying business is going to take?" Such statements may or may not reflect an interest in discussing PAS. Exploration of such statements may help clarify whether patients are simply tired and asking about prognosis or whether they wish to discuss with you possible hastening of death.

Here, we should pause for definitions. PAS can be defined as the intentional hastening of death performed by a person with decision-making capacity with the assistance of a physician (and other clinicians). Voluntary euthanasia is defined as an act intended to hasten death performed by someone else (usually a physician) with the permission or at the request of the person. (Involuntary euthanasia would be hastening death without the consent of the person.) At the present time in the United States only PAS is legal and only in Oregon under specific circumstances.

No one on either side of the PAS debate worthy of respect advocates a simple yes–no response to questions such as these. Even if you are sure you would never act with the intent of hastening a patient's death, do *not* start with a response such as, "No, I can't. It's illegal (or wrong)." *Do not overreact* to inquiries by dying people. I suspect that it is the rare individual who knows he or she is dying who has not at least considered the possibility of "getting the show on the road." Therefore, it is a mistake to assume such inquiries are the equivalent of active suicidal ideation and require an emergency psychiatric consultation and the placement of a hold for "danger to self or others." Neither should you underreact with a response like, "Oh, you don't mean *that*, you've got plenty to live for" or by ignoring a sometimes subtle, sometimes not so subtle request to discuss the issue.

Most requests I have encountered that might be interpreted as requests for a hastened death incorporate some ambiguity. Some, such as the question, "I want to die, can you give me something," are relatively unambiguous, although it is still not clear what the patient wants in requesting "something." "Will you help me when my time comes" may have nothing to do with a hastened death. The patient may simply be asking will you help me (be there) when my time comes (when I die). Hence, clarification of such ambiguity is helpful. This can be as simple as "What do you mean by 'help you when your time comes,'" but usually it requires deeper exploration of what is being requested and the context and understanding within which such a request is being made.

To the extent that an individual requests a hastened death, an exploration of that person's story is strongly advised. A variety of questions can be asked:

Why are you asking about a hastened death?
Why are you asking right *now?* (The timing of a request is rarely accidental. The timing may reflect a new pain or worry or might represent a patient feeling more comfortable with you as a clinician in raising a difficult issue that has been on his or her mind for some time.)
What factors might be influencing your thinking?
  Pain or other distress, either current or feared in the future
  Concern about being a burden
  The cost of continued care and associated monetary loss
  Fear of loss of self-control
  Depression or other psychic distress[37]
What do you think will happen to you if you do not have a hastened death? (For example, one patient with bony metastases who had little pain said he assumed that all his bones would break and result in unspeakable agony.)

How might a hastened death resolve your concerns?

Have you discussed your thoughts with important people in your life?

   If not, why not?

   What do they think?

   What are they struggling with—how might a hastened death affect their lives?

How would you make sense of a hastened death relative to the rest of your life?

What role do you imagine I or other members of the health care team should have in all this?

Although posed as a series of questions, in reality the discussion should be a dynamic exchange. The clinician may comment on specifics (such as your bones will not all break) and empathize and respond to questions posed by the patient (or family member). None of these questions will be of much help if you cannot establish a supportive atmosphere and demonstrate real concern and empathy with the person's situation.

Using the GOOD Acronym and Requests for PAS

The GOOD acronym may help you explore a request for PAS. Key ingredients— identifying stakeholders, determining the person's goals, discussion options (including alternatives to PAS), and exploring values are all relevant. At some point you will have to offer your opinion and, beyond this, clarify your bottom line in terms of what you can and cannot do. However, the reader is cautioned not to jump ahead to his or her bottom line but to see a request for PAS as an opportunity to explore how that person wants to live the rest of his or her life. Such discussions are not so much events or tasks as processes of engagement with patients struggling mightily with very difficult decisions.

Pronouncing the Patient[38,39]

"By the power invested in me by the State of California, I pronounce you dead." I do not know if a physician has ever actually said these words, but I have heard the tale of the "pronouncing resident" several times. A resident shows up at the door of a patient whom he has been called to pronounce. The family is grieving at the bedside. The resident may ask the family to leave the room while he performs the ceremony. In one variation the resident calls out this pronouncement from the doorway. Although I hope this is just a myth, it would not surprise me at all if it were true. The very sad fact is that most physicians learn nothing about how to pronounce a patient during their years of clinical training. They may watch a more senior resident do it once or twice or may follow instructions from a handbook, but they never actually receive training.

Why include a section on death pronouncement in a chapter on communication? After all, the patient is usually, well, dead. The issue in death pronouncement is less "diagnosing death" than it is acknowledging the passing of a human being and helping grieving loved ones. The ritual of death pronouncement requires exquisite communication skills on the part of the clinician. Family and loved ones in their grief turn to the physician for consolation. Just as families remember how a birth is handled, so, too, will they long remember how a death is handled. This will be one of the most important moments in the lives of survivors. Beyond this, like birth, if any time in the lifecycle is sacred, it is this time.

When called to pronounce a patient, if the patient is unknown to you, first inquire about the circumstances of the death. Was it expected or not, traumatic or not? Inquire about the status of family and loved ones. Are they present or not? Did they expect the death or not? What does the caller know of their emotional state? Do they seem at peace, in shock, or angry? Such knowledge will help prepare you for notification and consolation of the family.

There is no established, "official" procedure for pronouncement. Technically, you must "certify" that the patient has died. This is usually the simplest part of the process. Death is an easy diagnosis. The first step in pronouncing a patient begins within you. This is a time to set aside other concerns, a time to focus. Try to find a calm and peaceful place within yourself before going to the bedside. It may help to pause for a moment outside the room to take a few quiet breaths, then enter the room respectfully with an open mind as to what you may find. If no one else is present, you can confirm that the patient has died and, in your own way, say goodbye. Confirming death is usually easy. In fact, in approaching most people who have died, it is obvious that they are dead. Many clinicians have shared this same experience—they cannot say exactly how they know, but they do. We can sometimes be fooled, so for confirmation and as a part of our medical ritual we tend to feel for a pulse, listen for a heartbeat, and watch for respirations. The lack of a pulse is not specific to death. People with low blood pressure frequently loose their radial pulse hours to days before they die. Prolonged periods of apnea, not breathing, and Cheyne-Stokes respirations can also be deceptive. People close to death may breath shallowly or intermittently, sometimes with pauses that last minutes. Examination of pupils is not important and may be seen as invasive by family members. Assessing response to pain or noxious stimuli, as some physicians have learned, can be incredibly offensive if done in the presence of family members and seems to me to be disrespectful of the deceased.

If family, friends, or other clinicians are present, watch for a moment and assess how they are handling the death. Some may already have acknowledged the death and be actively grieving. In such cases your main job is one of consolation. Others may not have recognized that death has come, or, more commonly, they may need your official confirmation that the person has died in order to acutely grieve. In the latter case I may listen with my stethoscope ritually (knowing that I will not hear breathing or heart sounds) before informing those present that the person is gone.

Sensitivity is necessary to assess the needs of those present at the deathbed. If people are actively grieving, we must bear in mind that this is an exceedingly private moment in which we are privileged to participate. Figuring out how to come "into sync" with acutely mourning families is most difficult. Sometimes families are engaged in very important rituals or are expressing their most personal thoughts. In such cases we must stand on the periphery and look for an opening for when they will need our assistance. In other cases there is an openness to the grief that invites participation. We are called to the circle to share and bear witness to a passing. Sometimes people seem to call out to us: "You, you doctors. You are the masters here. We are overwhelmed and on foreign soil. Help us find safe passage." Although we must acknowledge to ourselves that we, too, are on "foreign soil" and do not really understand what death is about, we must know when to take the lead.

For example, because the immediate grief reaction is so intense, there may be a tendency for participants to hurry the first few moments of acute grief. I recall a wife who was just beginning a great sob, when she pulled it all together, cut off her grief, and asked, "I'm sure there must be some forms for me to sign." While I try to avoid telling people how they ought to grieve, it seemed she was pushing away a part of herself that really wanted to wail for a few minutes, so I said, "There will be time for all that. I want you just to sit here for a few moments to let this all settle a bit." She accepted this lead and sat, letting her grief come.

There is a time in this process when words do no justice. I think of this as the "sacred silence." This silence opens a space in which the living join the dead, together in the mystery of life and death, becoming and unbecoming.

Usually families want some time to themselves after a pronouncement visitation. My hospice nurses have taught me some of their art of giving space while staying connected with families and loved ones during this private time, which may last minutes to hours. Our nurses remain highly alert, just on the edge of the family's space and awareness. They watch for a sign that this family time has passed and their assistance is needed. A family member may stagger toward the door with a "what do we do now" expression. Just then, usually with impeccable timing, our nurses are there to help guide them through the business at hand. This amazing dance between the nurses and the family tends to go unnoticed, yet it never ceases to fill me with admiration. If there were a scene I would like to be able to show people about what makes hospice different, it would be this one—a synchrony so perfect that I suspect families and outsiders do not even notice that something special is happening. It takes great skill and compassion to do something so special that it seems to be nothing special.

When calling a family member at home to notify of a death in the hospital or nursing home, different skills are required. Physicians dread having to call people to notify them of the death of a loved one. This is particularly awful if the death is unexpected by the family. Sometimes this cannot be helped. Some people die with absolutely no warning. More often, I believe, families could be made aware that death is imminent if clinicians were more skilled in recognizing the signs of impending death. Too often families are not informed of this by clinicians, which unnecessarily compounds the shock of the phone call.

Especially if the death is unexpected by the recipient of the call, this is usually a "bad news" episode of communication. The reader may wish to review the steps in sharing bad news and consider how these steps might be modified, given that the news is not being shared in person. Consider that the person may be completely unprepared to receive bad news. You are not in control of the setting in which the news is being received. You cannot assess nonverbal communication nor show empathy with body language. You do not know who else is on the other end of the line. Given all this, it is obvious that sharing bad news by telephone stinks, but sometimes we cannot help it.

When calling to notify someone of a death, it is often difficult to assess what the recipient's understanding was of the deceased's prior condition, but it is worth trying to figure out. Will this phone call be expected or not? Getting an unexpected telephone call, especially at an awkward hour, usually implies bad news, so the introduction and advance alert should be brief. Having given the news, it can be very difficult to judge reactions over the telephone. If wailing is heard, what does that mean? You may ask questions about what is happening—who is there, what are people doing. People tend to ask a barrage of questions on the telephone. It is usually best to give only simple, short answers and let the other person know that you can discuss things in more detail at the hospital (or wherever the death happened). A common mistake is to ask the family member to come to the hospital *right away*. In fact, there is no hurry, and acutely distraught people can be a safety hazard on the road. Inquire whether someone is with the person or if someone can come to the hospital with the family member.

I do not think this is common practice, but it makes sense to me to give the name of a contact person at the hospital (or nursing home) for the bereaved person to ask for upon arrival. Acutely grieving people need to keep things very simple and personal. That person may be you, the caller, but may be someone else, after a change in shift, for example.

I remember being called by the nursing home when my father died. We were told to come in "right away." We knew my father was dying and suspected this was what had happened, but we were never really told. With my brother and mother, I headed for the nursing home. As we approached the nursing desk, the nurses seemed to huddle closer to one another. "Here they come, the Hallenbecks!"—they seemed to be whispering. Being the physician–son, I took the lead in approaching my father's room. In my heart I already knew Dad was dead before opening the door. He was gone. We grieved, and we were OK. However, it occurred to me later that what had happened was not OK. People should not have to "find" their fathers dead. People should not have to try to locate someone who knows something about their dead loved one when they come to the hospital or nursing home. People should be told to connect with a particular person who can guide them into the presence of the deceased and offer assistance as needed.

Follow-Up

If you had a close relationship with a patient and call to offer your condolences a few days later, such a call is almost always highly valued by family members. Indeed, this is considered exceptional for a physician, above and beyond the call of duty. Even if you do not personally call, it seems it should be the minimum standard of care that someone from your healthcare organization call, at least as a courtesy. You might also consider writing a condolence letter.[40]

Pronouncing a patient and consoling the bereaved immediately following a death is hard work. To do it well takes energy and great attention. If we are truly empathetic, we will encounter deep emotions such as sadness, anger, and despair, all while we are overwhelmed with other tasks and often sleep deprived as well. Pronouncing a patient reminds us that we, too, are mortal. In the faces of the deceased we may see reflected our grandmothers, grandfathers, parents and even ourselves. Clinicians may feel guilty: If only we had done this or that, then perhaps he or she would not have died. In addition, we may feel angry over the circumstances of the death. We may feel trapped by a system and a society that has not come to grips with dying. Often, we feel helpless. If you have such feelings, it only proves that you are still human. Clinicians also grieve. You may need to take some time out following a pronouncement. Even a few minutes outside in a garden may refresh you. If you are really struggling with some issue that a death raises for you, consider finding someone you trust to talk to. As a profession of healers, we do a terrible job of supporting and healing one another.

In touching death we experience a common humanity that transcends our roles as clinicians. None of us understands much about death, but in bearing witness to the passing of a fellow human being, our humanity is affirmed. In this we can all find solace.

Summary

Of the various skills needed in palliative care, none is more important than the ability to communicate effectively. Without such skill, little else is possible. Unfortunately, no skill tends to be so taken for granted. I have also found no area to be more challenging educationally. Our fast-paced medical world demands that things be neat and tidy—crisp, bulleted presentations at noon conferences over pizza. Such approaches work poorly for subjects better learned through apprenticeship and informal learning. However, I have also found no area more fascinating, challenging, and rewarding. Nothing is more delightful than to connect with a patient or family member and, often suddenly, come into mutual view. Having found each other, we can share a cup of tea and tell some stories.

References

1. Hahn, R. *Sickness and Healing—An Anthropological Perspective*. 1995, Yale University Press: New London, Conn, pp. 164–72.
2. Beckman, H. and R. Frankel. The effect of physician behavior on the collection of data. Ann Intern Med 1984; 101: 692–6.
3. Waitzkin, H. Information-giving in medical care. J Health Soc Behav 1985; 26: 81–101.
4. Good, B. and M. Good Delvechio. Patient requests in primary care clinics. In: N. Chrisman and T. Maretski, eds. *Clinical Applied Anthropology*. 982, D. Reidel: Boston, p. 287.
5. Tulsky, J. A., M. A. Chesney, et al. How do medical residents discuss resuscitation with patients? J Gen Intern Med 1995; 10(8): 436–42.
6. Tulsky, J. A. et al. Opening the black box: How do physicians communicate about advance directives? Ann Intern Med 1998; 129(6): 441–9.
7. Billings, J. A. and S. Block. Palliative care in undergraduate medical education. Status report and future directions. JAMA 1997; 278(9): 733–8.
8. Covinsky, K. E. et al. Communication and decision-making in seriously ill patients: Findings of the SUPPORT project. The Study to Understand Prognoses and Preferences for Outcomes and Risks of Treatments. J Am Geriatr Soc 2000; 48(5 suppl): S187–93.
9. Roter, D. L. et al. Experts practice what they preach: A descriptive study of best and normative practices in end-of-life discussions. Arch Intern Med 2000; 160(22): 3477–85.
10. American Association of Medical Colleges. The increasing need for end of life and palliative care education. Contemporary Issues in Medical Education 1999; 1–32.
11. Buss, M. K., E. S. Marx, et al. The preparedness of students to discuss end-of-life issues with patients. Acad Med 1998; 73(4): 418–22.
12. Huddleston, D. and R. Alexander. Communicating in end-of-life care. Caring 1999; 18(2): 16–8, 20.
13. Quill, T. E. Initiating end-of-life discussions with seriously ill patients: Addressing the "elephant in the room." JAMA 2000; 284(19): 2502–7.
14. Siegler, E. L. and B. W. Levin. Physician–older patient communication at the end of life. Clin Geriatr Med 2000; 16(1): 175–204, xi.
15. von Gunten, C. F., F. D. Ferris, et al. Ensuring competency in end-of-life care—Communcation and relational skills. JAMA 2000; 284(23): 3051–7.
16. Shorr, A. F. et al. Regulatory and educational initiatives fail to promote discussions regarding end-of-life care. J Pain Symptom Manage 2000; 19(3): 168–73.

17. Good, B. *Medicine, Rationality, and Experience: An Anthropological Perspective*. 1994, Cambridge University Press: New York, pp. 65–87.

18. Broyard, A. *Intoxicated by My Illness*. 1992, Clarkson Potter: New York, p. 53.

19. Suchman, A. L. et al. A model of empathic communication in the medical interview. JAMA 1997; 277(8): 678–82.

20. Hallenbeck, J. A Dying Patient, Like Me. Am Fam Physician 2000; 62: 888–90.

21. Hallenbeck, J. L. and M. R. Bergen. A medical resident inpatient hospice rotation: Experiences with dying and subsequent changes in attitudes and knowledge. Journal of Palliative Medicine 1999; 2(2): 197–208.

22. Rappaport, W. and D. Witzke. Education about death and dying during the clinical years of medical school. Surgery 1993; 113(2): 163–5.

23. Hafferty, F. and R. Franks. The hidden curriculum, ethics teaching and the structure of medical education. Acad Med 1994; 69(11): 861–71.

24. Rabow, M. W. and S. J. McPhee. Beyond breaking bad news: How to help patients who suffer. West J Med 1999; 171(4): 260–3.

25. Buckman, R. Breaking bad news: Why is it still so difficult? BMJ (Clin Res Ed) 1984; 288(6430): 1597–9.

26. Buckman, R. *How to Break Bad News*. 1992, Johns Hopkins University Press: Baltimore.

27. Quill, T. E. and P. Townsend. Bad news: Delivery, dialogue, and dilemmas. Arch Intern Med 1991; 151(3): 463–8.

28. Ptacek, J. T. and T. L. Eberhardt. Breaking bad news. A review of the literature. JAMA 1996; 276(6): 496–502.

29. Ambuel, B. and M. Mazzone. Breaking bad news and discussing death. Primary care: Clinics in Office Practice 2001; 28(2): 249–67.

30. Ptacek, J. T. et al. Breaking bad news to patients: Physicians' perceptions of the process. Support Care Cancer 1999; 7(3): 113–20.

31. Hallenbeck, J. L. What's the story—How patients make medical decisions. Am J Med 2002. 113(1): 73–4.

32. Braddock, C. H. III et al. Informed decision making in outpatient practice: Time to get back to basics [see comments]. JAMA 1999; 282(24): 2313–20.

33. Meier, D. Should it be legal for a physician to expedite a death? No: A change of heart on assisted suicide. Generations 1999; 23(1): 58–60.

34. Coombs Lee, B. Should it be legal for physicians to expedite a death? Yes: What experience teaching about legalization of assisted dying. Generations 1999; 26(1): 59–60.

35. Lee, M. A., L. Ganzini, et al. When patients ask about assisted suicide. A viewpoint from Oregon. West J Med 1996; 165(4): p. 205–8.

36. Drickamer, M. A., M. A. Lee, et al. Practical issues in physician-assisted suicide. Ann Intern Med 1997; 126(2): 146–51.

37. Breitbart, W. et al. Depression, hopelessness, and desire for hastened death in terminally ill patients with cancer. JAMA 2000; 284(22): 2907–11.

38. Marchand, L. R., K. P. Kushner, et al. Death pronouncement: Survival tips for residents. Am Fam Physician 1998; 58(1): 284–5.

39. Weissman, D. E. and C. Heidenreich. Fast Fact and Concept #4: Death pronouncement. End of Life Education Project. http://www.eperc.mcw.edu/, 2000.

40. Menkin, E., R. Wolfson, et al. Fast Fact and Concept #22: Writing a condolence letter. End of Life Education Project. http://www.eperc.mcw.edu/, 2000.

9

Working the System and Making a Difference

We must become the change we want to see
Mahatma Gandhi, 1869–1948

A medical student with whom I had worked went to study palliative care in London. During her stay she was fortunate enough to meet Dame Cicely Saunders, founder of the modern hospice movement. She returned from her studies and was anxious to tell me of her visit with Dr. Saunders. "We spoke of various issues and problems in palliative care in the United States—insurance, the Medicare Hospice Benefit, medical education, and the like. Dr. Saunders said to me, 'Well, why don't you change things?' Exasperated, I replied, 'What do you want me to do, Dr. Saunders, become the president of the United States?' Dr. Saunders quickly replied, 'Why, that would be a lovely idea!' Dr. Hallenbeck, she really suggested that I become the president!"

This story tells us something about the legacy Dr. Saunders leaves for us. The modern hospice and palliative care movement became a reality because Dr. Saunders and her successors identified problems and then set out to solve them. The student who met with Dr. Saunders had emigrated from Vietnam as a child refugee. She was a third-year medical student at the time of their meeting. Given our country's history, it borders on the absurd to think she might become president—but it did not so seem to Cicely Saunders. The message Dr. Saunders delivered to a visiting student and to the rest of us is to appreciate our potential to effect change regardless of our current stations in life and to encourage us to act on that potential.

When I think about all the problems in modern health care, I tend to become depressed, angry, and discouraged. As one comes to understand the magnitude of change that will be required to deliver truly excellent palliative and end-of-life care for patients, it is easy to become overwhelmed, to give up and wait for others to act. It is true that major changes must occur in the underlying structures of how care is delivered and reimbursed. It is also true that our society has a long way to go in coming to grips with serious illness and how we die. Educational deficiencies abound for health care professionals and the lay public. It is tempting to think, "Perhaps someone smarter, more energetic, or more powerful than I will be able to solve these problems." Perhaps this will happen, but then again, perhaps not. Maybe it is up to us to make a difference.[2,3]

When I attend on the general medical wards in our hospital, on the first day I have begun asking the team members, resident, interns, and medical students why they decided to go into medicine. They tend to speak of the great intellectual challenges involved in diagnosis, treatment, and research, yet behind these words one can hear that virtually all are driven by a simple desire to be of help to others. When I reflect this observation back to them, they nod sheepishly in agreement. I suggest that when they find themselves getting angry at others or frustrated during the month, they consider that other people are also doing this work because they, too, wish to be of help. I am encouraged that this underlying spirit of helpfulness lives on, often despite an otherwise dehumanizing medical system. If we can tap into this spirit, then there is hope.

During such attending months I am amazed at the inventiveness of the teams in "working the system." Residents take great pride in knowing exactly who to talk with in order to expedite a certain test or procedure. An ability and willingness to work the system can have a major impact on patient health care outcomes. The problem is that the extent of the system clinicians are so skilled in working is largely restricted to the inpatient hospital and to a lesser degree outpatient clinics. If we consider what the relevant "system" is for seriously ill and dying patients, we can see how restricted this clinician universe is. Home care, nursing home care, and community support, all critical system elements, are largely ignored in medical curricula or, at best, given token acknowledgement. For too many hospital based clinicians, when patients and families leave the grounds of the hospital, they are on their own, sucked through a black hole into some parallel, very alien universe from which they occasionally and mysteriously reappear in emergency rooms. To the extent clinicians can expand the scope of their concern and interest in working the system to include patients' entire universes, they can significantly improve their ability to be helpful.

Even within the hospital setting, the efforts of house staff are too often restricted to getting *around* the system rather than changing the system for the better. While their motivations for going into medicine may have been noble, the grinding work of residency training forces them to focus as much on their own survival as on excellent care for their patients.[4] Getting patients the care they need melds with an overpowering drive to expedite the processing of patients so the "service" does not become overloaded. It almost seems too much to ask trainees who are struggling with survival and the care of individual patients to broaden their scope and consider changing the system itself. Somewhat paradoxically, in order to empower house staff and other clinicians to change the system for the better for their patients, we must improve the system for clinicians as well. To the extent clinicians can rise above "survival mode," they may find the needed energy for changing the system on behalf of their patients.

Medical education has not stressed the importance of systematic change as a means of promoting health. Young physicians have come to believe that a good doctor is a knowledgeable doctor.[5] The doctor who can cram the most facts into his or her head is the superior physician. Clinical skills, both cognitive and procedural, are also highly valued. It is worth noting, however, that historically the greatest effect on health and mortality worldwide resulted not from clinician knowledge or skill, but from systematic changes in sanitation, which preceded not only the discovery of antibiotics but even modern germ theory.[6,7] In recent years the notion of public health, focused more on collective well-being than the health of the individual patient, has atrophied to near nonexistence.*

Given all this, it is a wonder that positive change in the system happens at all. Fortunately, there are always a small number of people who understand the great importance of improving the system. Although Cicely Saunders was right in suggesting that we should set lofty goals for ourselves, I am sure she would agree that one does not have to become the president in order to make a significant contribution. This book is written for the serious student of palliative care. Clinicians who find their way to palliative care are highly motivated to be of help to patients and families. They cannot help but become aware of how flawed the current health care system is. Here I am suggesting that simply becoming clinically competent in the provision of palliative care, important as this may be, is an inadequate response to the suffering around us. Each of us, regardless of our position, must work to change the system for the better.

Someday I hope a good history of hospice and palliative care will be written. The story is full of heroes (and remarkably few villains). I have had the privilege

---

*In the United States at the time of this writing, public health is witnessing a resurgence in interest in large part in response to the September 11th attack and a new awareness of the risk of bioterrorism.

to know some of the leaders in palliative care, and their work and commitment are truly inspiring. I have been equally inspired by the work of many individuals working at local levels. Let me share one example.

A group of second-year Stanford medical students came to recognize that their preclinical training on topics related to palliative care was seriously lacking. Stanford has a course in the second year called Preparation for Clinical Medicine (PCM), a well-designed course used to jump-start students for their clinical training. These students developed a half-day course on communication—how to share bad news and discuss goals of care—and got this into the PCM curriculum. It was a wonderful thing to see—three second-year medical students teaching a group of faculty, including two associate deans, how to act as facilitators for this course. The course has been positively received. The students went on to publish what they did in a special issue of *Academic Medicine* dedicated to end-of-life care.[8] As any medical school faculty member can tell you, there is nothing harder to change in medical school than is the curriculum. How did these students accomplish this? Beyond their obvious dedication and precocious understanding, their great strength lay in the fact that they were *students*, not faculty who were advocating for change. Faculty members who push for curricular reform are suspect because expansion of vested interests is often viewed as turf-building. The students could not be so accused. Their interest in changing the curriculum was selfless, and they were right to point out deficiencies. To Stanford's credit, the medical school deans listened to the students and were willing to let the students lead the way. At least sometimes there is an advantage to being the little guy.

I have begun to a collect a list of interventions that might be accomplished through the initial work of one individual, although it is not comprehensive. Some interventions are clearly of larger scale than others, some requiring the cooperation of a number of individuals. Some require only a single committed person. Some examples have already been undertaken by individuals and groups, and some are at this point only ideas, as far as I know. The key point is that just as there is always something you can do to help an individual patient, so, too, there is always something that can be done to improve the system of care. My hope is that this list will stimulate readers to try something out, whether it is on this list or not, and to share their actions with others.

Education Initiatives

- Develop talks, handouts, and laminated cards.
- Share your work with others. For example, you might submit your curricula to the End of Life Physicians Educational Resource Center at http://

www. eperc.mcw.edu. Submitted educational material will be peer reviewed and listed on their Web site, allowing you to make this material available to others.

- Obtain a dedicated slot in your organization's conference schedule for topics related to palliative care.
- Evaluate the educational content offered in your facility for the percentage and quality of palliative care content.
- Sample the available textbooks in the library, the chief resident's office, and clinic offices. How many of these have quality palliative care content? If there is no other way to get it, *buy* a good textbook on palliative care and donate it, conspicuously, to an area actually used by residents.
- Feed back collected information to important change agents—clinic chiefs, residency program directors, department chairs, and so on—with kudos for those doing good work and suggestions for areas that might need attention.
- Model conducting literature searches for questions related to palliative care on the computer in the resident call room. Bring in palliative care articles to the ward team regarding symptom management that result from your search.
- Add major palliative care websites to favorite/bookmark lists for computers with internet access, such as Growth House at http://growthhouse.org—the major connection point for virtually everything relating to palliative care on the net.
- When hearing presentations on research with possible implications for palliative care, ask specific questions: How were quality-of-life issues addressed in the study? How do researchers think this new finding might result in less suffering?
- Do a small study or review of a palliative care issue. Present this at a conference or submit it for publication.
- Work to incorporate palliative care issues into existing educational forums. Examples are residents reports, ICU rounds, morbidity and mortality conference, clinic teaching sessions, and grand rounds.

Symptom Management

- Review your hospital formulary's commonly used palliative medications. Advocate for those medications that have a special niche in palliative care.
- Assess how symptom assessment and management is included or not included in notes and care plans by physicians, nurses, and other clinicians.
- Target a specific intervention, such as using subcutaneous rather than IM shots of morphine, increasing the use of long-acting opioids for chronic pain, and the barriers to proper opioid use caused by local policies that actively discourage use, such as frequent renewal policies.

- Address common practices based on little, if any, data that may be harmful, such as chronic use of meperidine and the use of lorazepam as a sole agent for nausea.

Decision Making and Communication

- Take a stand on assessment and documentation of patient preferences. Set standards for yourself and those you supervise. If you are an attending or resident physician, what do you expect to see on the history and physical charts regarding patient preferences? What do you say to your subordinates? Is documentation of preferences a good idea, an option, or an expectation?* Do you model this? How important is such documentation relative to other data you would expect to see, such as an examination of the heart and lungs?
- Have specific skills included on a sanctioned procedure check-sheet for residents. What skills might be listed? Sharing bad news, pronouncing a patient, notifying family, addressing prognosis. . . . ?
- Model these skills to those you supervise.
- Make brochures and documents, such as durable power of attorney and out of hospital DNR forms, available in key areas, such as clinics.

Psychosocial Issues

- Do an assessment of the resources available to support patients and families in your community, such as disease-specific support groups and ethnic support groups.
- Identify useful websites that can help patients and families with special needs and give them to patients during clinic visits.
- Learn about special transportation systems, such as volunteer groups and special elderly transportation systems, that get patients and families where they need to go.
- Identify bereavement support in your community both for routine and complicated bereavement.

---

*My own practice when attending on the wards is to require "an intelligent note" on preferences before attending rounds on all patients. Often, housestaff do not initially take me seriously. When I point out the lack of an intelligent note, they usually protest: "It seemed like a bad time to chat—he was exsanguinating!" or, "He was demented without a family member present." The "curriculum" begins when we can discuss how to incorporate such eventualities into an intelligent note. For example, an intelligent note might state, "Patient is demented and family not available. Prior preferences not documented. Will attempt to contact tomorrow."

- Identify interpreters and cultural guides for your population and learn how you can access them. Make this available to others.
- Check for documentation of psychological factors in hospital and clinic notes, such as documentation of possible depression or delirium.
- Ask families of patients (especially in ICUs and nursing homes) to bring in a photo of what the patient looked like when well, and post it in a visible spot.
- Add a profile of who the patient was during morbidity and mortality conferences—a photo, video, statement, or poem to remind participants that the patient was more than pathologic tissue.
- Assess bereavement support in your facility, especially in areas when high-impact deaths occur, such as the ER, transplant units, and ICUs. Work with allies to establish a policy that the families of all patients who die in your facility receive a minimum of one bereavement follow-up call.
- Work with your billing office to ensure that once a patient dies, a bill is not subsequently addressed to the deceased.
- Rename your inpatient waiting room a "family room," then stock it so a family would want to be there, with toys, video tapes, books, and magazines that people might actually want to read. Get staff or volunteers to donate kids' videos and used books to the room. Make it a matter of ward staff pride to create the most homelike family room in the facility.
- Obtain a portable CD or tape player and ask staff to bring in old CDs and tapes that patients or families might enjoy.
- Start a "video legacy" program. Get a video camera and a tape recorder (for those patients who would rather not be remembered looking ill). Offer to tape messages and other communication that can be sent to family members who cannot visit the patient and to leave a valued memory for the family.
- Buy a stack of telephone calling cards that can be given to patients and families in need to enable them to make important long-distance telephone calls.
- Abolish "visiting hours."
- Develop a system to accommodate families of dying patients who are keeping a vigil in the hospital. Where can they sleep—roll-away cots? Can they order a tray of food to be delivered to them?

Spiritual Issues

- Identify resources for spiritual assistance for your patient population.
- Place telephone numbers and lists of clergy in easily accessible places.
- Find reference books for patients and families who request help with spiritual support.

- For patients who cannot see, obtain audiotapes of major religious texts that they can listen to.

Venues of Care

- Invite members of agencies with whom you work to come to teach you what they can offer.
- Identify key contact people within agencies with whom you work. Invite them to talk with your group about how you might better serve the patients you share.
- Set up listserve/email links between people at different venues to facilitate communication.

Awards

- Give awards to those allies who are just beginning to do something new. Special achievement awards can be created for house staff, ward teams, your clinic nurses—anyone who has made a special effort related to care. (It does not take much effort to print a unique special award document on a computer.)

Making a Difference in a Moment

Anything you do that can be experienced by more than the individual with whom you are working can make a difference simply by modeling good behavior.

- Model treating a severe symptom, such as pain, as a medical emergency.
- Model spending as much time (or more) with a dying patient as with a patient who has a fascinating diagnosis.
- Model finding a chair and sitting down when making rounds.
- Model listening.
- Speak up politely but firmly when people say something such as, "He's just here for pain control." "He's just an old guy dying." "She's a social admission." "He's just here for placement."
- Make a statement regarding your priorities to those you supervise and to your supervisors: "Working to provide good care at the end of life is a priority for me." "I'm trying to document carefully patient preferences for all seriously ill patients." "There *are* more important things than placement." "Trying to provide excellent symptom management is as important to me as is getting the right diagnosis." "I keep trying to see the person behind the patient behind the disease."

Most great acts of history began with the actions of one individual. The challenge, it seems, is for the individual to engage those around him or her, to strike a resonant chord and thereby find allies in a common cause. Clinicians really want to be of help, and we all know in our hearts that we have a vested interest in good care; at some point almost all of us will require it for those we love and for ourselves. This is our strength. If we can engage this common interest in better care for the seriously ill and dying, one can become many.

References

1. Kalish, R. The aged and the dying process: The inevitable decisions. In: J. Carse and A. Dallery, eds. *Death and Society*. 1977, Harcourt Brace Jovanovich: New York, pp. 301–12.
2. Lynn, J. and J. Schuster. *Improving Care for the End of Life: A Sourcebook for Clinicians and Managers*. 2000, Oxford University Press: New York.
3. Lynn, J., S. Meyers, et al. Fast Fact and Concept #44: Changing the status quo. End of Life Education Project. http://www.eperc.mcw.edu/, 2001.
4. Addison, R. A grounded hermeneutic editing approach. In: B. Crabtree and W. Miller, eds. *Doing Qualitative Research*, 2nd ed. 1999, Sage: Thousand Oaks, Calif., pp. 145–61.
5. Shorter, E. *Bedside Manners*. 1985, Simon & Schuster: New York.
6. Rosenberg, C. *The Care of Strangers—The Rise of America's Hospital System*. 1987, Basic Books: New York.
7. Golub, E., *The Limits of Medicine—How Science Shapes Our Hope for the Cure*. 1994, Times Books: New York.
8. Magnani, J.W., M.A. Minor, et al. Care at the end of life: A novel curriculum module implemented by medical students. Acad Med 2002; 77(4): 292–8.

10

Palliative Care Consults

"She says, if you please, sir, she only wants to be let die in peace."
"What! And the whole class to be disappointed, impossible! Tell
her she can't be allowed to die in peace; it is against the rules of
the hospital!"
  John Fisher Murray (1811–1865) *The World of London*

Palliative care consults are a relatively new phenomenon, at least in American
hospitals. A handful of articles have been published to document the tasks to be
performed and some outcome measures of the consultation process.[1-6] Very little
has been written on how to actually do a palliative care consult.

In performing consults we face an interesting challenge—how do we incorporate the principles and practices of palliative care into a highly ritualized form
of interaction that has evolved within the world of traditional medicine? That
the consultation process is so ritualized is a mixed blessing. On the one hand,
consults as a method of interaction are very familiar to clinicians; assuming the
role of a consultant may make it easier for others to accept what we have to
offer. On the other hand, palliative care clinicians may feel like "strangers in a
strange land," constrained by some rituals that seem quite alien to good palliative care practices. Understanding the implicit rules (and tensions) in the consultative process and how they may affect our work is a necessary first step.

In the hospitals within which I have worked, a major tension exists between two different models of consultation. One model stresses *giving advice* to the primary physician or ward team, and the other stresses *taking over* some aspect of care. The latter approach appears to be more frequent in tertiary academic hospitals and where discrete technical skills (such as the ability to perform endoscopy) are required. General internists and family medicine physicians tend to prefer the advisory role, when possible, which keeps them in the loop. Many subspecialists, at least in academic medical centers, prefer the take-over role, even when working at a nontechnical discussion phase of consultation. For example, most oncologists I know, when consulting in hospital on a patient with a new diagnosis of cancer, minimally involve the ward team in decisions regarding options, such as chemotherapy and radiation therapy. After all, what does a general internist know about these options? This frequently gives rise to resentment on the part of primary care physicians, who will readily admit that they are not experts in oncology but who may think they have something to contribute in terms of understanding the totality of the patient. Similarly, many cardiology consultants, when asked their *opinions* about whether cardiac catheterization is advisable, will go ahead and schedule catheterization, if thought appropriate, without discussing this with the primary care team.

My experience is that neither model is ideal for palliative care consults; a good consult requires a delicate blend of approaches. For example, ward teams may wish for us to take over certain tasks, such as talking with patients and families about care options, but would be offended if we discussed certain medical treatment options with which they might not feel comfortable. For example, I have recommended dexamethasone for a patient with pain due to a compression neuropathy. However, the primary care team, worried about immunosuppressive side effects, did not want to take this recommendation. Had I mentioned the medication to the patient, this would have put the primary care team in an awkward position. An additional problem for palliative care consult teams is to figure out to what extent education of other clinicians is a task they wish to undertake. Educating clinicians can add time to the consultation process and cut down on efficiency. However, a major objective in performing consults should be to educate clinicians in what palliative care has to offer and help them to incorporate palliative care into their own practices.

Modeling certain skills to primary care team members, such as discussing preferences, can be an efficient and effective way of teaching skills. Of course, this requires coordination in the timing of meetings with patients and families, and it is time consuming for the observing team members. When possible, however, this is a superb way to help other clinicians understand what we do, and skill development is promoted.

Because palliative care consults are a relatively new phenomenon in most hospitals, many referring clinicians will be unfamiliar with what we have to offer.

Some clinicians will be opposed to the whole idea of such consults. Naïve unfamiliarity is apparent when clinicians do not know when it would be appropriate to request a palliative care consult. Thus, many patients who could benefit from a consult do not receive it, or they receive it later than would be ideal. Because our consult team is associated with an inpatient hospice unit, most of the "consults" we obtained in the months following the establishment of our team were merely requests for transfer to our hospice ward. Although not bad per se, such consults reflected a mind-set in which consultation was solely about *placement* at a time when the primary care team had decided this was appropriate. Such requests do not acknowledge a helping role for the consult team, other than by getting the patient "off the service." Clinicians often mistakenly believe that palliative care consults are restricted to patients who are overtly terminally ill, if not imminently dying, and who have decided on comfort care only. "Active therapy" with life-prolonging agents is too often understood as a contraindication to a consult. Thus, for example, when a patient had a completely obstructed esophagus due to cancer that resulted in a distressing build-up and overflow of saliva, his team initially thought that the fact that he was to receive chemotherapy and radiation therapy contraindicated a palliative care consult. (At least they called us, asking if it was appropriate to obtain a consult. We assured them that it was. We advised a slurry of glycopyrrolate to dry up salivary secretions followed by artificial saliva. This was very helpful to the patient.) The rarest type of palliative care consult we receive is for nonterminal patients who have difficult symptoms the primary care team cannot adequately address. An example was a consult for a patient with pruritus (itching) secondary to an impacted gallstone in the common bile duct pending endoscopic removal.° Based on our experience, there is no easy fix for such unfamiliarity. Distributing flyers and giving presentations on "what palliative care consults can do" can help, but gaining trust and understanding is a long, slow process.

More difficult is dealing with frank hostility to palliative care consults. Hostility can come both from clinicians and from patients and families. Naïve hostility often arises from simple misunderstandings. Well-intended clinicians may inform a patient or family that the "hospice group is coming to talk about stopping therapy and going to a very nice place to die." As one patient who had received such advanced billing put it when we first met, "So you're guys who are going to pull the plug on me!" Clinicians (and patients and families) may resist consults because they may come to symbolize evidence of the patient's

---

°Notably, cholestatic pruritus is not mediated via histamine receptors. Thus, the clinicians, who tried antihistamines, had no success in treating his itching. This form of pruritus involves pain fibers and responds best (if opioids are not being used, as was the case here) to naloxone. Naloxone administration in this case resulted in instant and near complete relief of his itching. A slow naloxone infusion was maintained until the stone was removed, which resolved the underlying problem.

deteriorating, often terminal, clinical course, which may be difficult to face. Some will be actively hostile to consults if and when they believe the consult will result in a negation of their current or proposed care plan. At times palliative care consult teams are drawn into a battle without even knowing it. For example, it is not rare in my experience for primary care clinicians to argue with oncologists over whether a patient should receive aggressive chemotherapy. Without even knowing it, a consult may represent an invitation to engage in ritual battle with oncologists. To the extent we are viewed as "reinforcements" in such a battle, we should not be surprised to encounter hostility. A little advance scouting can usually determine if and when we are being set up for such a battle.

More subtly, we may encounter resistance from groups with whom the discipline of palliative care overlaps. A consult request to palliative care may be considered unnecessary because specialists believe they *ought* to be able to handle the issues at hand. In being identified as specialists in a particular domain of care, physicians come to believe they should know everything about patient care that in any way relates to that domain. The sad fact that most such specialists have received little training in palliative care as it relates to their particular disciplines does not assuage their belief that they ought to be competent in all aspects of care related to their specialty. Thus, the oncologist believes that he or she ought to be able to provide *all* care related to a cancer patient. The pulmonologist thinks that he or she ought to know how to treat *all* forms of dyspnea, and the cardiologist is of the opinion that he or she must be an expert on *everything* related to congestive heart failure. Our involvement in the care of their patients may be seen as an affront to their expertise.

The greater the overlap between palliative care and other specialties, the stronger yet less obvious this resistance can become. For example, geriatricians, who overlap greatly with palliative care in their work with chronically ill and dying elders, may overtly view palliative care practitioners as allies in a cause serving such patients (as we are). However, they may be slow to recognize the need for palliative care services for geriatric patients distinct from the care they provide, thinking that they ought to be able to provide such care for elders based on their credentialing, even if their training was deficient in specific palliative care skills. Similar resistance can be found among pain management specialists, who may view palliative care consults as competition. Early in our process of establishing a consult team, we found, somewhat to our surprise, that some general medicine attending physicians became quite irate at finding us talking with their patients. We would inform them that their resident team had requested the consult. "Well, *I* was not informed of this!" was the reply. Although one would think this was an intraward team problem of miscommunication, I doubt the same attending physicians would have been offended to find an infectious disease consultant at the bedside of a patient with an exotic infection, as they would readily acknowledge the specialist's expertise. At least in our hospital, residents often request consults without first informing the attending physician. So what was going on? I think these very good physicians felt that in discussing certain things such as goals of care and preferences we were infringing on their areas of expertise (working with the whole patient) and thus felt an affront. We have since built in the step of ensuring that the attending physician is aware of the consult before we perform it.

In summary, palliative care consults exist in a politically charged environment. Consults must address these political concerns if they are to be accepted and the team is to be successful.

Many consult requests also are emotionally charged. Except for very straightforward consults such as for a hospice referral or for treatment of an isolated physical symptom, most consults occur in an atmosphere of desperation. Commonly, a major disagreement arises between some involved parties, and help is needed to resolve such conflict. These emotionally charged issues usually exist in the subtext of a consult request. The consult may state, "Instruct patient and family about the dying process," when what is really going on is, "The patient and family are driving us crazy. They keep requesting therapies that will not work. We've tried to explain to them that the patient is dying, but they just don't get it. I hope you palliative care people have some magic tricks up your sleeves so that you can get through to them." Identifying this emotional subtext as it applies to clinicians, patients, and families is usually a key task in the consultation process.

Performing Consultations

As suggested above, most consults are not straightforward requests for advice regarding a particular symptom but rather very difficult processes of communication and relationship building in emotionally charged situations. Thus, most critical to performing consults is skill in communication. The GOOD acronym— identifying goals and options, giving one's opinion and then documenting the consult—is a useful way to think about performing a consult. Here, I highlight key tasks within this general structure and indicate how the GOOD structure may be modified to accommodate the consult process.

1. Identify stakeholders. The people who request the consult are the most obvious stakeholders in the process. Of course, we hope patients and families will also be involved and will benefit from our work. Other consultants, case managers, and discharge coordinators are often other key stakeholders.
2. Identify overt and covert issues in the consult. Almost always, certain problems are overt in a consult. The team may be requesting transfer, help with a symptom, or assistance with communication. These are usually easy to identify. More difficult to identify are covert issues—unstated, often emotional issues on the part of consult requesters and others. Often, these must

be teased out from conversations with key stakeholders. For example, in the case of Mr. C, discussed at the beginning of Chapter 8, I first talked with the ICU team members. When they told me that if something was not done soon they would have to insert a tracheostomy and a feeding tube, I said something like, "My, that must be worrisome"—a form of empathetic mirroring. "You bet it is worrisome! We don't want to do *that*," was the reply. In consulting on a case of a "simple" hospice referral in which oncologists are involved, I might ask, "What do the oncologists think about the patient going to hospice?" "That's the thing," comes the response. "The oncologists just refuse to recognize that he is dying. They are pushing for an experimental treatment. You know how they are." Oh, so the covert request is for assistance in dealing with the oncologists. The sooner we know this, the better we will be able to respond.

3. Identify the stories. Different stakeholders often have very different stories—especially when related to an emotionally charged issue of dispute. As highlighted in the GOOD acronym, it is usually helpful to inquire as to stakeholders' understandings of what is going on. In talking with stakeholders and reviewing the chart, the consultant should try to piece together these stories, looking for points of convergence and divergence. In battling with an oncologist, the primary care team's story may be that the patient is dying and that the oncologist cannot see this and is overall too aggressive. Discussion with the oncologist may reveal that she does recognize that the patient is dying, but the patient keeps asking if any experimental therapy is available because she is not ready to give up. Reluctantly, the oncologist feels obliged to offer such therapy. As these examples illustrate, stakeholder stories go beyond that particular person's opinion of the patient's medical status and wishes regarding a preferred option to include their perceptions of other stakeholders' stories. The primary care team's story incorporates a perception of the oncologist's story. The oncologist's story incorporates an interpretation of the patient's story and tries to make sense of a request for experimental therapy.

A chart review, in addition to providing important medical data about the patient, can be very revealing of certain aspects of clinicians' stories. Histories and physicals (H&P), discharge summaries, and progress notes can be notable not only for what they say, but also for what they do not say. Too often, the H&P and initial progress notes make little, if any, reference to a patient's goals of care, or symptomatology. The patient, as a person, is rarely revealed. Often, the only clues to psychosocial issues, goals of care, and subsequent venues of care are to be found in the case manager, social worker, or discharge coordinator notes, not the physician or nursing notes. If the patient's situation is not improving, short references at the end of notes often suggest that clinicians are growing concerned or frustrated. Usually, there is a clear precipitant to the request for a consult, which should be sought by the consultant. The precipitant is usually helpful in understanding the timing of the request and may hint at covert issues. For example, a utilization review note that pushes for discharge may hint at many possible tensions. Why is the patient still in the hospital? Is discharge a reasonable option? Is there some tension among clinicians, patient, and family as to posthospital options? Have care alternatives even been addressed?

4. Clarify roles. Different stakeholders are likely to have different expectations (overt and covert) about your role as a consultant. In hearing clinician, patient, and family stories, it is often necessary to clarify the consultant's role, especially when the consultant's perception of his or her role differs from that of a stakeholder. If, for example, the primary care team wants the consultant to "do battle" with another consult team, the consultant should clarify that, while the consult team owes the requester an honest opinion, it does not engage in battles. With patients and families it is particularly important to emphasize that our only goal is to be helpful. So often in a conflict, patients and families come to believe that we are there to talk them into something they do not want to do. An explicit statement of "neutrality" is very helpful, although such a statement may not initially be believed. I often say, "I am not here to talk you into anything. My only goal is to be helpful to you, your family, and the care team." In saying this or similar words, the consultant must truly *be* neutral and not attached to any particular outcome. In giving an opinion to clinicians, patients, or family, one might say something such as, "I owe you my opinion. However, whatever you choose to do with it is entirely up to you." One cannot even become attached to the goal of performing a *successful* consult, however that might be defined.* Such neutrality, combined with a sincere statement of one's intent to be helpful, often puts people at ease. I have also noticed that consultants who make such statements become calmer, an infectious condition that serves the process well. The words I use, as in the above example, speak more of neutrality, as this is usually easiest for clinicians, patients, and families to understand. Neutrality, as I am using the term, does *not* mean without passion or commitment. I may care very deeply about what is happening and have a strong opinion as to what might be best to do. What I really mean in talking of neutrality is not investing oneself in particular outcomes. In interacting with others and in offering my

---

*As palliative care consults become more popular in the hospital because of success with difficult problems or patients, unrealistic expectations can arise as to what the team can do. Showered with praise, consultants may drive themselves toward repeated success. Consultants may judge their work a failure if, for example, a patient rejects all overtures to establishing a relationship. Working for "success" can create a quiet desperation in the consultant, which poisons the consultative process.

opinion, I try to commit myself completely to the process and to be clear in my opinion. However, having done so, I cannot invest in such things as whether the advice is taken.

5. Identify options. In hearing clinician and patient stories, certain options become apparent. Very often, consults are precipitated by a clear disagreement about options, such as whether to go to hospice. Just as often, certain options will not be apparent to clinicians or patients. Such options may include where to live under what conditions or may concern management of a particular symptom. If the consultant identifies an option that is either not apparent to a stakeholder or that has already been flatly rejected, attempting to make sense of it in relation to that person's story is a key task. A case may help clarify this point.

At the beginning of this chapter, I mentioned a patient who said to our team, "So you're guys who are going to pull the plug on me!" This was Mr. S. Let me share a little more of his story. Mr. S had advanced small cell carcinoma of the lung. Three rounds of chemotherapy had had no effect on his tumor progression. Although the oncologists were "considering" a fourth round, their hearts were not in it. Mr. S had been a loner for many years and had lived in a trailer. He hated being sick but hated losing control of his situation even more. Communication among the ward team, the oncologists, and the patient had deteriorated to the extent that he ordered them all out of his room whenever they visited. They had mentioned hospice as an option, but that just made him more upset. When the intern called for the consult, she said, "Don't tell him I called you. He already hates me!" In response to the above greeting, I told Mr. S that our only intent was to help and that we were not there to pull the plug or to push for anything. "How do you think you are doing," I asked. "Like shit," he replied. He then needed to tell us of all the ways the doctors and nurses did not listen to him, lied to him, and controlled his life. We sat quietly and listened. "That sounds miserable," I responded. "Where do you think you are headed from here?" "I just want to go home to my trailer and be left alone." It was clear to us that Mr. S had an "external locus of control"— that is, he externalized the causes of his problems. At the same time, he desperately wanted to be in control of everything—a sure-fire recipe for suffering. It was also clear that Mr. S hated being on an acute medical ward, which for him epitomized lack of control. We first explored the possibility of where he might live outside the hospital. He admitted that, for now, the trailer was out, as he needed more help than that would allow. He had a daughter, but she worked and went to school full time. He did not want to impose. His estranged wife had even offered to let him live with her, but he nixed that idea, "That's out." Then we began exploring institutional options other than the acute ward. They were effectively limited to three choices—a regular nursing home (which he refused), a rehab-oriented ward, and our inpatient hospice ward. We explored the advantages and disadvantages of the rehab and the hospice wards. In discussing the hospice option, to which he was initially allergic, I said, "I want you to listen for a moment to what the hospice ward has to offer. Just forget about the H word for a minute. . . ." Mr. S also had a number of distressing physical symptoms. I explained that our staff was more skilled in addressing these symptoms than was the rehab ward. Because self-control was such an important issue to Mr. S, I also highlighted the fact that the hospice ward was less restrictive in terms of letting him live as he wished, including the possibility of allowing passes to visit family. In short, I discussed the two ward options in terms of his story. Only after this did we explicitly discuss hospice philosophy and his goals of care. As it turned out, he was not opposed to a palliative approach, he just wanted to keep his options open, and, as is often the case, he needed reassurance that it was fine not to give up hope. In fact, we told him we wanted him to be hopeful. We did *not* push hospice as an option. As the consultant, I had to be accepting if he rejected this advice and chose the rehab floor or to be discharged to his trailer, even though I believed both would be very foolish choices. The next day we met with his daughter. She and her father toured the unit, and he decided to be transferred. The day following his admission to our unit, he said, "I should have come here a long time ago!"

6. Give opinions. As mentioned in the section on the GOOD acronym, an opinion should be clear regarding what is being recommended and on what basis. To the extent possible, opinions should take into account the stories of the involved stakeholders and the facts as they are understood. They should relate to points of disagreement and should work to bring different story lines together. In the case of Mr. S, I clearly stated that I believed his needs would best be served on our unit. However, I assiduously avoided trying to convince him of this.

As discussed above, in thinking about offering an opinion the consultant must first consider what aspects of the opinion should be given to the patient or family and what aspects should be offered to the ward team or attending physician. In giving an opinion (recommendation) to the ward team or attending physician, make sure the overt questions asked in the consult have been addressed. If the consult says, "Please evaluate patient for appropriateness for hospice," make sure this is commented on. More covert issues are often better responded to informally. Usually, there will also be numerous aspects of care that the consultant thinks could be improved on. The patient may be on an inadequate laxative regimen. The breakthrough opioid dose may be insufficient relative to the basal dose. Artificial saliva might help with the patient's dry mouth, and so on. In addressing such specifics, the consultant should prioritize a few key recommendations, at least initially, regarding such care but should avoid trying to make things "perfect" with a laundry list of suggestions. The reasons for this are threefold. First, too long a list of suggestions risks overload. The ward team or requestor might implement some but might omit the most important suggestions. Second, the subtext to the recommendation may be interpreted by the requestor as, "You do not know what you are doing and are a terrible doctor. That is why I have to give so many recommendations." Third, a cardinal principle for all consults is *help* more than you *hurt*. That is, while you may ask the requestor to do certain things, such as change some orders, on balance the requestor should perceive that you are decreasing his or her work rather than increasing it. The help:hurt ratio can be favorably adjusted by offering to do certain recommended tasks yourself. For example, when recommending home hospice you could help by offering to contact the hospice, if this is agreeable to all parties, rather than recommending that the requesting team do so.

Giving recommendations and opinions often involves giving feedback on care that has already been provided. The recommendations we give often involve suggestions that the requesting team do something different, and thus, in effect, feedback is given that earlier care was less than ideal in some way. In giving feedback a simple but effective technique is to use the "sandwich" approach. First, go out of your way to give positive feedback: "Its great that you have him on a laxative while giving morphine. That is so often forgotten about." "I was happy to see you using a long-acting opioid for his pain." "The patient told me how much he appreciates your care." Then, give recommendations and negative feedback: "However, using just a stool softener is usually not enough when someone is on morphine. Most people need a promotility agent, like senna." "However, the Vicodin you have prescribed is at too low a dose relative to the basal opioid dose." "I noticed that nobody on the team addressed the patient's goals of care during the first two weeks he was in hospital. For a patient with advanced disease, I think this is a priority. Perhaps if the goals had been addressed earlier, it would have saved a lot of trouble." Finally, try to end on a positive note: "This was a great consult. Thanks so much for thinking of us." "It's clear the team has been working very hard to try to help this patient. I know it has been a struggle for you. You deserve a lot of credit for hanging in on such a difficult case."

7. Document the consult. Documenting the consult in the medical record is a necessity but often seems anticlimactic to the consult process. I recommend that the consultant think carefully about what needs to be written and what could better be handled informally. For example, you might recommend adding senna every evening for constipation. You might informally give the

feedback that DSS is an inadequate laxative in discussing the case with the intern in order to save face for the intern. Documentation is a useful way both of summarizing what has happened and of giving explicit recommendations. My notes usually summarize in story form my understanding of the current situation, areas of disagreement, overt questions posed in the consult request, and my overall impression. I then list, in ritual consult form, recommendations. You may also provide some education in the chart by explaining, for example, why a certain medication is recommended, taking care not criticize other clinicians. You might even give the team a short handout that discusses the issues at hand. Because it is difficult to express uncomfortable emotions such as anger or frustration in person, it may be tempting for some to try to express such feelings through the chart. This should be avoided. Because we are human, we will sometimes get upset, but it is far better to deal with these emotions, especially as they relate to other clinicians, off-line and in person.

Summary

Performing palliative care consults is challenging and rewarding work. It is amazing to me that the availability of palliative care consults is more the exception than the rule in most hospitals. I believe that in the not distant future palliative care consult teams will become routine. I look forward to a time when palliative care consults and the widespread provision of palliative care are nothing special, just part of a continuum of healing for the patients and families we serve.

References

1. Bascom, P. B. A hospital-based comfort care team: Consultation for seriously ill and dying patients. American Journal of Hospice and Palliative Care 1997; 14(2): 57–60.
2. Weissman, D. E. Consultation in palliative medicine. Arch Intern Med 1997; 157(7): 733–7.
3. Abrahm, J. The palliative care consultation team as a model for palliative care education. In: R. K. Portenoy and E. Bruera, eds. Topics in Palliative Care. 2000, Oxford University Press: New York, pp. 147–60.
4. Bruera, E. et al. Edmonton Regional Palliative Care Program: Impact on Patterns of Terminal Cancer Care. CMAJ 1999; 161(3): 290–3.
5. Nelson-Marten, P., J. Braaten, et al. Critical caring. Promoting good end-of-life care in the intensive care unit. Critical Care Nursing Clinics of North America 2001; 13(4): 577–85.
6. Homsi, J. et al. The impact of a palliative medicine consultation service in medical oncology. Support Care Cancer 2002; 10(4): 337–42.

11

The Final 48 Hours

For all flesh is as grass, and all the glory of man as the flower of
grass. The grass withereth, and the flower thereof falleth away.

I Peter 1:23–24

The old woman sat quietly in the corner of a darkened room watching her son,
who lay dying on the bed. He had colon cancer. She had breast cancer. His turn
came first. I could not imagine what it was like for her, a dying mother with a
dying son. I wondered if she saw a reflection of her own impending death before her. She was peaceful but curious. Perhaps, living herself in death's shadow,
this dying did not seem so alien and her son not so far away. I sat next to her,
and we watched together silently. Roger lay deep upon his mattress, but there
seemed to be a lightness about his spirit that was new since the day before. His
breathing slowed a bit and then sped up. There was a soft, purring sound, somewhat like a cat but not quite the same. When he breathed, his mouth opened
slightly. His face was relaxed with eyes half opened. He looked . . . not asleep,
not in a coma, not quite here anymore yet not yet gone either. "I guess he's getting
close," she said. I nodded. "Doesn't look so bad, does it?" "No," I said, "it doesn't
look so bad."

One thing is certain: each of us will have a last 48 hours. For some a final stage
of dying will be recognized, while for others death may come as a complete sur-

211

prise. For those who do "take a turn," as hospice staff say, a pathway is entered that has many common features.

This phase of dying, variably called the "terminal phase" or "active dying," is characterized by a series of changes that affect the dying person, the family, and clinicians.[1] For many dying patients this phase seems almost anticlimactic. They enter a dreamlike state and seem to progress peacefully in their dying. Some do have a hard time, and we need to know how to help them. Families often struggle mightily during this period. Clinicians are also seriously challenged. Few have been taught about active dying. Most lack even basic competencies. Clinicians are humbled before death as it becomes so obvious at a certain point that we are not in charge at all.

Lay people would be amazed if they knew how little clinicians know about active dying. They mistakenly think, "You see lots of patients die, you must know what this is about." However, in my experience the greatest lack of clinical knowledge in palliative care exists in this area. Dissecting cadavers in anatomy may teach clinicians about dead bodies, but it teaches nothing about dying. In a study by Merlynn Bergen and myself that examined the experiences of internal medicine residents who rotated onto our hospice ward, interns reported feeling the least knowledgeable about the physical changes of dying.[2] I suspect their experience was something like mine as a resident. I was too busy looking at numbers—lab values, vital signs, O_2 saturation monitors, and so on—to pay much attention to how people died. I am not sure that I ever simply sat with a dying patient. My patients either "coded" or were found dead with a DNR status. I do not remember many patients who died. Even now, although I have cared for many dying patients, it is a rare privilege to be able to sit with patients when they actually die. At one level there is a mystery to dying that defies explanation or rational understanding. The closer I am to death, the more aware I am of how little I understand about it. I suppose I should be patient—I will find out eventually. Given these limitations, what we can say about active dying can only be told from the very biased perspective of one who is not actively dying. However, we must start somewhere.

Predicting Active Dying

We have learned the most about active dying from following cancer patients, because their dying trajectories tend to be the most predictable. However, patients with other disease processes can certainly enter a pathway largely indistinguishable from that of cancer death. Morita identified four signs that heralded impending death in 100 cancer patients: the "death rattle," respiration with mandibular movement, cyanosis of the extremities, and lack of radial pulse. He measured the median time to death from the onset of these signs. They tended to occur in a rather orderly fashion, with the death rattle preceding respiration with mandibular movement (74% of the time), which in turn preceded cyanosis and pulselessness (63% of the time). The median time until death following the death rattle was 23 (+ or − 82, SD) hours, 2.5 (18) hours following respiration with mandibular movement, 1.0 (11) hours following cyanosis, and 1.0 (4.2) hour following lack of radial pulse.[3] (I was struck by this study because until I read about mandibular movement, I had been unable to see it in my dying patients.)

As this study suggests, many patients who are actively dying have "noisy respirations." These sounds come from retained secretions in the pharynx and the upper respiratory tree. Sometimes called terminal pneumonia, it is unclear how often such secretions represent true bacterial pneumonias compared to retained normal secretions in patients who are no longer able to cough.

This terminal syndrome, as we might call it, is easiest to identify in solid tumor cancer patients and is usually preceded by a bedridden status and little, if any, oral intake of food or fluids. The patient rarely speaks, or speaks only in brief phrases. A weak cough may be present initially but then disappears. The respiratory rate is variably increased and often becomes irregular, sometimes with frank Cheyne-Stokes respirations. The stethoscope is of minimal use. The buildup of respiratory secretions in the bronchi and bronchioles makes localization of underlying alveolar involvement, manifested by rales, difficult, if not impossible, to detect. More useful is direct palpation of the chest wall for vibrations that represent the buildup of secretions, a form of fremitus. If such vibrations occur only in the center of the anterior chest over the trachea, this may reflect only tracheal secretions and generate a false positive finding for active dying. These may subsequently clear if cough returns. However, peripheral fremitus appears to be more suggestive of terminal retained secretions. Fever is often absent, particularly if steroids have been used. The pulse may be strong initially but becomes threadier and eventually will not be palpable as blood pressure falls. Despite the lack of fever, peripheral vasodilatation may occur if there is underlying sepsis. In such cases the pulse initially is rapid and often hyperdynamic, which can be erroneously read as a "strong pulse." Most likely, this pulse results from a widened pulse pressure, because enhanced cardiac output under adrenergic stimulation is accompanied by a fall in systemic vascular resistance, especially if sepsis is present. I have found that feeling the shins for warmth is useful in evaluating for this. Because the shins have poor vascularization and normally are cool (especially in the presence of hypotension with reflexive vasoconstriction), warm shins conversely suggest vasodilatation. (Note that the sensitivity and specificity of these suggested examinations have not yet been tested.)

Although further studies need to be done on the short-term prediction of dying, I have found these signs useful but not infallible. Some patients with obstructive lung disease, those prone to chronic aspiration such as stroke, and dementia patients may rattle with retained respiratory secretions and yet not be actively dying. Cyanosis and mottling of the *upper* extremities appear more specific for impending death than do such changes in the *lower* extremities, where they commonly reflect peripheral vascular disease. I have witnessed false positives for mandibular movement in patients who have obstructive lung disease. The exaggerated use of strap muscles in breathing may result in jaw movements that mimic true respiration with mandibular movement. I suspect this sign in dying people results from relaxed muscular tone in the jaw combined with deep breathing. This might explain additional false positives I have seen for this sign in patients with benzodiazepine overdoses and amyotrophic lateral sclerosis (two patients each in my experience), both situations that involve relaxed muscular tone.°

A common mistake I have made and witnessed in others who work in hospice is to inappropriately extrapolate from cancer to other illnesses in predicting active dying. Most cancer patients do seem to follow a common dying trajectory, and hospice workers become quite good in recognizing when cancer patients enter the active dying phase. Mistakes occur when clinicians excessively extrapolate from this experience to other illnesses. In Chapter 2 I discussed "sinewaving," a vacillating dying trajectory in which patients with certain illnesses such as congestive heart failure and dementia may deteriorate and then improve— over and over again. For sine-waving trajectories, it is more difficult to state definitively that any given clinical deterioration will, in fact, lead to death.

Clinicians may also fail to predict the deaths of patients for a different reason—the tendency for patients with certain illnesses to die relatively suddenly. Obviously, patients at risk for catastrophic events such as cardiac arrhythmia or exsanguination may die suddenly and unpredictably, although relatively few such patients are followed in hospices. The more common mistake in hospice relates to patients at risk for sudden respiratory failure. Such patients are characterized by a lack of any respiratory reserve. Patients with severe intrinsic lung disease such as obstructive lung disease and pulmonary fibrosis are at risk for this trajectory. Less obviously, those patients who lack respiratory reserve because of neuromuscular disorders such as amyotrophic lateral sclerosis or Guillain-Barré syndrome often die suddenly and unpredictably. My guess is that in such

---

°To my knowledge, this little-known sign of active dying has been studied only in cancer patients. While many people sleep with their mouths open, commonly called the "O" sign, sleeping patients do not usually exhibit this gentle opening and closing of the mouth. Having watched for this sign for several years, my impression is that it is a relatively specific sign, if present, for active dying, but that it lacks in sensitivity. The few false positives I have observed were in patients with profound neuromuscular weakness and, occasionally, chronic obstructive pulmonary disease (COPD) as described in the text. The cause of this finding is unknown, but based on these observations, I suspect it results from *incomplete* relaxation of the facial muscles. If fully relaxed, as in REM sleep, the mouth does not move. This suggests to me that while there are similarities between dreaming and active dying, important differences, as yet unstudied, also exist.

patients who lack respiratory reserve, any pulmonary "insult" such as a mucous plug, food aspiration, bleeding, or early pneumonia is enough to tip the balance toward CO_2 retention and sudden death.

I stress this point because I have generally found it helpful to explain to families (and some patients) the possibility or probability that we may *not* be able to predict impending death for patients with such illnesses. If, in fact, such a patient is found dead, family shock seems dampened by foreknowledge of this possibility. Although some may be disturbed to learn of the inherent uncertainty in predicting such deaths, many are relieved to learn that active dying will not be drawn out and that most such deaths seem peaceful. Patients who suffer from severe baseline dyspnea, as do most such patients, tend to be more terrified of worsening dyspnea and suffocation than they are of dying. They are often quite relieved to be informed that the active dying phase is likely to be very short— measured in minutes to hours, rather than days.

Symptoms of Active Dying

Many people do fine during active dying. However, certain symptoms may arise that require attention.[1,4-6] In a study of symptoms that occurred in 200 actively dying cancer patients, Lichter found the symptoms shown in Table 11.1.[7]

This study provides a useful checklist for symptoms to consider and some interesting food for thought. It is not surprising that incontinence was present in one-third of patients. The clinician may be surprised at the relatively high incidence of urinary retention. Clinicians may be fooled into thinking that lack of urine output reflects dehydration or renal failure. Palpating the bladder and watching to see if the patient is distressed and reaches for the groin may provide clues to occult retention. Nausea tends to fade in the actively dying, which is probably related to decreased oral intake. The percentage of confused patients

TABLE 11.1. Symptom Frequency (in percent)

Noisy and moist breathing	56
Urinary incontinence	32
Urinary retention	21
Pain	42
Restlessness and agitation	42
Dyspnea	22
Nausea and vomiting	14
Sweating	14
Jerking, twitching, plucking	12
Confusion	8

in this study seems remarkably low to me. The considerably higher percentage of restless and agitated patients suggests that altered states are not uncommon in actively dying patients. This begs the question of how one might distinguish "confusion" from "restlessness and agitation."

Actively dying patients frequently develop irregular, or Cheyne-Stokes, respirations.* Irregular breathing is rarely distressing to patients. Dry mouth persists far into the dying process and requires meticulous attention. Agitation or terminal distress can be very troublesome and often requires some degree of sedation. (See section on altered states in Chapter 7.) There is no evidence that such sedation (or treatment of pain with opioids) significantly hastens death in the last 48 hours, as Morita and colleagues found in a study correlating time of death with opioid and sedative doses over the last 48 hours.[8] Pains certainly were not rare in the Litcher study. New pains were identified 29.5% of the time. However, *no* pains were judged as persistent or severe. The study was conducted on a hospice ward. This stands in sharp contrast to the SUPPORT study, in which 50% of dying patients in the hospitals studied were judged by relatives to have had 7 of 10 or greater pain in the last three days of life.[9] In the Litcher study, 91% of patients were on opioids, and 91.5% of deaths were judged to be peaceful. This study is good news for those patients, families, and clinicians who want data regarding dying. Contrary to common fears, paroxysms of pain and great distress are uncommon at the very end. Most dying can be peaceful if we support it properly. Ellershaw and colleagues recently documented, using a standarized evaluation instrument, the Integrated Care Pathways (ICP) assessment tool, that 80% of the 168 patients followed had either good control of the three symptoms that were followed (pain, agitation, and respiratory secretions) or only one episode "out of control" in the last 48 hours when good palliative care was provided. "As death neared, there was a statistically significant increase in the number of patients whose pain was controlled."[6]

---

*Cheyne-Stokes respirations refer to a rhythmic change in respirations wherein breathing becomes shallower and shallower variably with a slowing in respiratory rate that culminates usually in complete cessation of breathing for several seconds to more than a minute. This is followed by progressively stronger respirations that become exaggerated and quite deep. This pattern is thought to result from abnormal brainstem responses to CO_2 levels in the blood—initially undercompensating and then overcompensating. Cheyne-Stokes respirations can occur in other nonterminal disorders such as heart failure and stroke. It is interesting to note that patients who are able to speak generally say that no distress is associated with this breathing pattern. From this we may extrapolate to dying patients, who usually cannot speak with Cheyne-Stokes respirations, and presume that the syndrome is not disturbing to the patient. However, family members and clinicians may assume or project distress into this syndrome and thus often need to be coached. I usually explain that the pattern results from a breakdown in "cycling" between the lungs and the brain and that, as far as we know, it is not bothersome to the patient. This can also be an opportunity to discuss that at some point breathing will not just pause, but stop altogether, marking the death of the person.

Treatment

Perhaps the biggest problem in the treatment of the terminal syndrome of retained respiratory secretions is an inappropriate extrapolation from nonterminal, bacterial pneumonia by both clinicians and families. Although both processes involve the lungs, they are radically different in their pathophysiologies and treatment; what is very appropriate therapy for one may be very inappropriate for the other. Usually, this terminal syndrome is not an isolated process but merely the tip of an iceberg. As the body begins to shut down, widespread organ dysfunction develops. The accumulation of respiratory secretions in the lungs (with or without bacterial pneumonia) is just one of the most visible and audible signs of systemic breakdown.

It is often important to explain to family members (and other clinicians) how this syndrome differs from nonterminal pneumonia. The latter can be viewed as an accident, or at least a complication of some other illness. The body attempts to fight in nonterminal pneumonia. The immune system aggressively responds, and the body tries to cough out the offending organisms. It is reasonable and appropriate to deal with such an invasion by attacking the invading organism. Hydration by IV may help maintain blood pressure until the battle is won and can aid in sputum production, which is useful in promoting a productive cough. Antibiotics assist the body's immune system to fight invading bacteria. Success means a return to baseline health. In the dying process, it is usually impossible to separate what is happening in the respiratory tree from the larger process of dying. Even if life were to be prolonged for a short time with therapies such as antibiotics (which may be perceived as benefit or burden), the patient will *not* return to a baseline of reasonable health. The patient is still dying, and life prolongation is usually transient, at best.

In this terminal syndrome it is my impression that IV hydration may result in increased respiratory secretions, although studies have not yet clearly demonstrated this to be true. Patients at this stage generally lack a cough. Increased secretions, if present, can be troubling—especially to family members, who are often bothered by the gurgling sound. Deep suctioning is usually futile, as secretions are present in the alveoli and distal bronchioles, not just in the trachea and bronchi. The suction catheter cannot reach these distal bronchioles, and cough may not be stimulated; little is suctioned out. While deep suctioning is discouraged, gentle suctioning of the oral pharynx may be helpful.

The broader use of antibiotics in palliative care is discussed elsewhere. Here it is worth pointing out explicitly that in this syndrome antibiotics are of limited value to the dying patient. (They may have symbolic or ritual value to the family or to clinicians.) In patients who are actively dying, there is no evidence that antibiotics significantly improve quality or quantity of life. If there is an effect, it is likely that antibiotics prolong life to a small degree. For some, prolongation of life by hours to days (if possible) may be a benefit and enable family members to visit and say goodbye. For others, such life prolongation may be considered a burden. If we took away the term 'antibiotic' and asked someone, "Consider that you are actively dying. You will probably die within 24 to 48 hours. I can give you a pill that may prolong your dying by a day or so with no great effect on your quality of life. Do you want me to give you that pill?" Many people would decline such an offer. Having said this, obviously we are not always correct in identifying patients as being imminently terminal. This is particularly true for patients with dementia, strokes, and obstructive pulmonary disease, as discussed earlier. One reasonable strategy for the use of antibiotics in patients for whom the goal of care is explicitly comfort only, is *not* to use antibiotics initially, but only if the patient rallies and begins to recover in the hope of speeding a return to baseline and thereby enhancing comfort. Such a "trial of antibiotics" may seem counterintuitive and is the inverse of how such trials are usually conceived, but it does make sense relative to the described goal of care.

I have suggested that traditional, or at least common, hospital responses to active dying, such as antibiotics and IV hydration, are of minimal, if any, help. Sadly, in palliative care we are often first put on the defensive by having to justify why we believe certain therapies will not help. However, we must not stop here. In fact, there is a great deal we can do to be of assistance to the actively dying and their loved ones.

Clinician Checklist for Actively Dying Patients

- Establish and maintain a peaceful environment.
- Notify and educate family about the possibility or probability of impending death.
- Review medications and other therapeutic interventions in light of the change in the patient's status. Are all the medicines being administered still necessary? Generally speaking, opioids and anticonvulsant medications should be continued, if possible.
- Adjust medication routes, as swallowing is likely to be lost.
- Consider adding a low opioid dose or increasing basal opioid by 25% if dyspnea is present or probable.
- If the patient becomes anxious, give an anxiolytic. If delirious, treat as described in the section on delirium in Chapter 7.
- Consider giving oxygen via nasal prongs or using a gentle fan.
- If respiratory secretions become troublesome, consider anticholinergic agents to dry them. Scopolamine 0.4 mg. S.C. q 4–6 h prn secretions is very effective. Scopolamine is highly sedating, which is often advantageous at this stage.

Atropine eye drops 1% (1–2 drops q1–2 h as needed) are often used in home hospice settings, where subcutaneous administration is difficult. Atropine is less sedating than is scopolamine and can overtly worsen delirium. An alternative agent, glycopyrrolate (1 mg PO or 0.1 mg parenterally TID), can be administered if one wishes to avoid sedation and delirium (as glycopyrrolate does not significantly pass the blood–brain barrier). Anticholinergic agents are likely to be more helpful if given early, as they prevent the production of secretions and do not remove existing secretions.[10] If hydration via IV or PEG tube is being given, discuss discontinuation, because further hydration may contribute to respiratory secretions.

- Occasionally, mouth suctioning of secretions can be helpful. Usually, deep suctioning is ineffective and unhelpful.
- Coach the family on the changes that are occurring (see below).

All of us need such reminders. (On more than one occasion, I have been politely approached by a nurse who was "just wondering" if I still really wanted a certain medication, such as a psychostimulant, given to an actively dying patient—a polite manner of suggesting that I should review medications.) However, the actively dying must not be approached mechanistically. Active dying is not a disease but a natural process that may benefit from support and facilitation. I recall a talk I heard by Tibetan Buddhist master Sogyal Rinpoche (author of *The Tibetan Book of Living and Dying*), who was discussing dying from a Buddhist perspective. He told us with a chuckle not to worry—we would all "die successfully." He was not suggesting that dying is necessarily easy or free of suffering, but he was warning us not to treat dying like some difficult final exam for which we have to cram in order to pass. It is my impression that while some suffering is engendered in dying for most people, this tends to fade in the active dying phase. Sometimes dying reminds me of a bad case of insomnia. People struggle with being sleepy while still being unable to sleep. Being caught between the conscious world and the world of sleep can be very unpleasant. However, when, finally, people do fall asleep, they usually do so totally. It is no longer a question of mind vs. body. Sleep, when it comes, is so obviously the right thing to do that no question or even consciousness of a question arises. The total person, body and mind, knows what to do; so, too, with dying. When people do die, they die totally and quite successfully. I find this very reassuring.

Who Is the Patient?

The phase of active dying often seems more difficult for families than for the dying themselves. Most people have never witnessed a death before. All sorts of fears, anxieties, and concerns well up and need to be addressed. Most of all, families need our support during this difficult, exhausting time. Families, loved ones, and even clinicians become the patients and look to us for support and guidance.

Elsewhere, I addressed concerns that commonly arise. It is common for families to question why more aggressive, invasive care is not being given: "Why aren't you using an IV?" "What about antibiotics?" "Shouldn't we move him into intensive care?" These issues may or may not have been already addressed, and even if they have been, second thoughts are common. Families, who have trouble accepting that dying is happening, may accuse staff of clinical errors or negligence. They can become very angry. When being accused of purposeful neglect or of knocking out Grandpa with morphine, it can be difficult not to overreact. It may help to realize that from the family's point of view, it is far easier to tolerate the idea of clinician error or incompetence than the fact that a loved one is dying. Both the cognitive aspect of these accusations (why we are not using an IV, etc.) and the affective component ("You seem very angry; it must be very hard seeing your loved-one like this") need to be addressed (see Chapter 8 on communication).

Coaching

One the most important methods of offering support to families (and others) during dying is coaching. Coaching involves a process of sharing knowledge and working with families as they practice new skills in a supportive environment. Coaching of families should parallel changes in the dying person. Changes are explained, and suggestions are made for how the families can adjust to them. I believe that such coaching allows families to better participate in the care of the dying, promotes comfort and peace for the dying, and helps families with their grief, which is transitioning from anticipatory grief to bereavement.

We can explain that the dying tend to let go of senses and desires in a certain order (with variations, of course, depending on the individual). First hunger and then thirst are lost. These losses usually precede the last 48 hours, and coaching is therefore also appropriate at earlier stages. Speech is lost next, followed by vision. The last senses to go are usually hearing and touch.

Palliative Care Note

The senses as well as hunger and thirst tend to be lost in an orderly fashion: first hunger, then thirst, then speech, then vision, then hearing, and then touch.

Families tend to frame their understanding of the loss of these senses and appetites in negative ways: "Look, she is starving to death." It may help to reframe the loss in more positive terms: "We don't really know why hunger and thirst are lost as they tend to be. One way to think about it is that she (the dying person) must let go of many everyday things in dying. People don't do this all at once. It is sad, but it is better than dying hungry or thirsty."

In addition to worrying about the dying person, family members are also grieving their own losses. Each of these losses of the senses and desires in the dying patient tends to be mirrored by losses in family members. Much of what seems to motivate families' concerns arises from this grief. For example, a loss of appetite and thirst in the patient tends to be mirrored by a grief reaction related to nurturing: "If I cannot feed or give fluids to my dying loved one, how can I nurture him?" We may explain the loss of appetite to families, but if they *hear* that we are saying they should not nurture the patient, they will rightfully reject our counsel. The question then becomes how can nurturing be transformed so that it will meet the needs of the family and be appreciated by the patient. Instructing the family that moistening the mouth or giving small sips of a cool liquid may be more appreciated by the patient than a large meal may help.

When speech is lost, otherwise alert patients may become frustrated by the inability to speak. Reassuring them that we understand their frustration and rewording our inquiries so they can be responded to with head nods or shakes (yes or no) can facilitate communication and reassure the dying. Families may need to be coached in these techniques. For families the loss of speech in the patient is mirrored by an inability to communicate in the usual way. What was for most families a two-way conversation becomes a one-way conversation, at least verbally. This, too, gives rise to grief: "How do I know what she is thinking or feeling?" Note that this question anticipates a much larger question for family members at this transition stage. What, if anything, will she experience when she is dead, and what will my relationship be to her? Families may think that patients who are unable to speak are unable to communicate, listen, or even be conscious. It is important to explain to them that many such patients can still respond and communicate nonverbally. At this stage we suggest that family members talk to the dying person in a peaceful, reassuring manner. I truly believe this helps most dying people, and most families have something important to say to the dying, such as "I love you."

I discussed my experience of "pronouncing" my own father's death in a nursing home in Chapter 8. His death occurred before I had become involved in palliative care. The night before he died I rushed across the country to see him. I entered his room, alone, as the doctor–son. He was breathing very rapidly, reflecting, I thought with my doctor's mind, some metabolic acidosis with a compensatory respiratory alkalosis. "Probably septic," I thought. His face appeared relaxed. I confirmed that he had received some morphine, and then I left. I saw him briefly the next day before he died. I deeply regret that I did not sit down and tell him what was in my heart. Whether he would have heard me

I do not know. I do know that doing so would have been good for me. What I needed was a coach to explain that he might be able to hear and to suggest that perhaps I sit with him, hold his hand, and talk with him. I needed permission to be a son saying goodbye to his father.

Some people, although not many, will ask what to say. I tend to answer, "What is in your heart," although a custom is emerging that there are certain parting words that should be spoken. Byock cites from a hospice nurse five "tasks" that may serve as parting words (although these tasks may better serve as a process among the dying, family, and friends at an earlier stage). These tasks are to ask forgiveness, to forgive, to say thank you, to say I love you, and to say goodbye.[11] These parting words may be shared in a two-way discussion or may form a starting point for families to speak to a dying patient at an advanced stage. It is important not to impose these tasks on patients or families, but they may be helpful for those searching for a starting point. I believe that these tasks may be carried out nonverbally as well as verbally.

There may be a brief stage in which the process of losing vision is troublesome to families. Patients may appear to be "looking right through you." This often feels spooky to families. The "look," as some hospice workers call it, is often accompanied by predeath visions. Patients at this stage may be on a different wavelength, as discussed in the section on altered states in Chapter 7. Families may project all sorts of meanings onto this look—"He's ignoring me or mad at me." It may help to explain this process (without necessarily trying to explain why, in fact, patients experience different wavelengths).

Most dying people then close their eyes and appear to be asleep. From this point on dying is very mysterious, and we can only infer what is actually happening. My impression is that this is not coma, a state of unconsciousness, as many families and clinicians think, but something like a dream state. Hearing and touch often seem remarkably preserved, suggesting some degree of consciousness. If people ask me how I know this, it is from the many cases in which a loved one, holding a dying person's hand, has said "I love you" and received a soft hand squeeze. In reassuring a dying person who has anxious respirations by saying "You are doing fine," the breathing pattern may slow and becomes peaceful. Families are thus encouraged to comfort their loved one with words and touch.

Clinicians may need to give family members permission to take a break from this final vigil. Some family members desperately perform a "death watch," believing it is critical to be present at the time of death. They may push themselves so hard that they threaten their own health. Basic needs such as eating and sleeping for those doing a vigil must be met. One may suggest that family members take turns. Because there is no way of knowing exactly when someone may die, it may be necessary to acknowledge that the patient might die during such a break. (Often such deaths are later interpreted in a positive light: "Joe was just waiting for me to leave in order to die. It was too hard with me there.") Most realize at some level that death has its own timetable. It may be helpful to suggest that as important as *physical* presence is and that being present at the moment of death is a great gift, love is not bound by time or space. Such coaching may also help survivors in bereavement, when the relationship with the deceased will not depend on physicality.

When Death Arrives

Death may arrive with a bang, but more often it comes quietly, without so much as a sigh. The moment of death is sacred in the deepest sense, and words do it no justice. It is a time to witness silently a passing. In bewilderment, some family members may become flustered and wish to begin too quickly all the formalities that follow death. I find it useful in such cases to remind family members that there is plenty of time for "arrangements" and suggest that perhaps they should sit for a while (see the section on death pronouncement in Chapter 8.) A natural time will come to begin the inevitable work that follows death—both the business of funeral arrangements and the work of grief. We watch for that moment by standing by and being ready to lend a hand when needed.

References

1. Abrahm, J. *A Physician's Guide to Pain and Symptom Management in Cancer Patients*. 2000, Johns Hopkins University Press: Baltimore, pp. 336–70.
2. Hallenbeck, J. L. and M. R. Bergen. A medical resident inpatient hospice rotation: Experiences with dying and subsequent changes in attitudes and knowledge. Journal of Palliative Medicine 1999; 2(2): 197–208.
3. Morita, T. et al. A prospective study on the dying process in terminally ill cancer patients. American Journal of Hospice and Palliative Care 1998; 15(4): 217–22.
4. Enck, R., *The Medical Care of Terminally Ill Patients*. 1994, Johns Hopkins University Press: Baltimore, pp. 161–72.
5. Conill, C. et al. Symptom prevalence in the last week of life. J Pain Symptom Manage 1997; 14(6): 328–31.
6. Ellershaw, J. et al. Care of the dying. Setting standards for symptom control in the last 48 hours of life. J Pain Symptom Manage 2001; 21(1): 12–7.
7. Lichter, I. and E. Hunt. The last 48 hours of life. J Palliat Care 1990; 6(4): 7–15.
8. Morita, T. et al. Effects of high dose opioids and sedatives on survival in terminally ill cancer patients. J Pain Symptom Manage 2001; 21(4): 282–9.
9. SUPPORT. A controlled trial to improve care for seriously ill hospitalized patients. The Study to Understand Prognoses and Preferences for Outcomes and Risks of Treatments (SUPPORT). JAMA 1995; 274(20): 1591–8.
10. Hughes, A. et al. Audit of three antimuscarinic drugs for managing retained secretions. Palliative Medicine 2000; 14(3): 221–2.
11. Byock, I. R. *Dying Well*. 1997, Riverhead: New York.

Afterword

Waxing and waning make one curve.

C. G Jung, *The Soul and Death*

Most people die as they have lived, for dying is part of living. If we wish to die better, we will need to learn to live better. If we reflect carefully on the deaths in which we participate, we will see much we wish to emulate and much we wish to avoid in our own dying. Such is the gift the dying offer. That people die is profoundly sad. In each encounter with death, this sadness acquires a new face. In sadness we can find a common bond of humanity. We find sadness and suffering, but not only this; we find peace and joy as well. Someone asked me once what it takes to do this job well. More than anything else, I think, it is the ability to enter deeply into the pain, suffering, and sadness that are a part of living and dying and then to emerge on the other side into peace and joy. Over and over again.

Index